Also by Karlis Ullis, M.D., and Greg Ptacek

Age Right: Turn Back the Clock with a
Proven Personalized Antiaging Program

Super "T"

The Complete Guide to
Creating an Effective, Safe, and Natural
Testosterone Supplement
Program for Men and Women

Karlis Ullis, M.D.

with Joshua Shackman
and Greg Ptacek

A FIRESIDE BOOK
Published by Simon & Schuster

FIRESIDE
Rockefeller Center
1230 Avenue of the Americas
New York, NY 10020

Copyright © 1999 by Karlis Ullis, M.D., Greg Ptacek and
Joshua Shackman

Designed by Pagesetters, Inc.

Manufactured in the United States of America

10   9   8   7   6   5   4   3   2   1

Ullis, Karlis.
    Super "T" : the complete guide to creating an effective, safe,
and natural testosterone supplement program for men and
women / Karlis Ullis, with Joshua Shackman and Greg Ptacek.
        p.   cm.
    Includes bibliographical references and index.
    1. Androgens—Health aspects. 2. Androstenedione—Health
aspects.   1. Ptacek, Greg.   II. Shackman, Joshua.   III. Title.
QP572.A5U45   1999
615'.766—dc21   99-14572
                                                             CIP
                    ISBN 0-684-86335-9

Acknowledgments

The authors wish to thank these individuals who made this book possible: the patients of the Sports Medicine and Anti-Aging Clinic who, wanting their lives renewed, were willing to try the newly available testosterone prohormones—the T-boosters; Harvey Klinger for shepherding the project through the obstacles of the publishing world; and Sydny Miner for her meticulous editing, advice, and support of the project at Simon & Schuster.

The authors also wish to thank these individuals for their important contributions to the book: Michael Mooney and Jim Brockman for sharing their wide experience and scientific expertise on the use of androgens (T-boosters and testosterone products) for building better lives and stronger bodies in HIV-wasted individuals as well as for their specific scientific insights; Cristiana Paul, M.S., for her nutritional proficiency and the many food tables, meal plans, and other valuable contributions found in Appendix 1; Shirley Kim and Preetpal Sandhu for their diligent research assistance; the administrative staff of the Sports Medicine and Anti-Aging Clinic, especially chief office administrator Yvette Harper and assistant Katherine Eisenhauer; Cheryl Woodruff for her editorial expertise; John J. Ullis for his never-ending computer technology support; and Harianto Harianto for data entry.

Thanks must also go to the medical doctors and scientists who have contributed so much to our current understanding of male hormones and their effect on both women and men: Shalender Bhasin, M.D. (his seminal research and publications showed what athletes have known for decades—super-high levels of testosterone do affect strength and muscle mass); Barbara B. Sherwin, M.D.; J. S. Tennover, M.D.; Ronald Swerdloff, M.D.; Christina Wang, M.D.; S. Davis, M.D.; Henry Burger, M.D., and Fernand Labrie, M.D.

Finally, a special thanks goes to Patrick Arnold, the innovative synthetic chemist who not only provided inestimable expert scientific advice but was also the first to develop and introduce to the consumer supplement marketplace most of the T-boosters discussed in this book. Without his new and novel testosterone prohormone supplement formulations, this book would not exist.

Contents

Contents

PART IV
Your Personal T-Booster Regimen

APPENDICES

Preface

It is my hope that this book is useful beyond informing consumers about the new class of prohomone supplements—T-boosters—and will also stimulate scientific interest in the emerging field of *intracrinology*. The term was coined by Fernand Labrie, M.D., who along with his coworkers in Quebec, Canada, initiated some of the first research into the physiology of prohormone transformations and related actions within specific tissue cell sites with their 1988 studies of DHEA.

Classically, endocrinology is about the levels of hormones in the blood and their effects on various tissues. The emergence of DHEA as a supplement prompted a rethinking of the action of hormones—away from the blood level model (endocrinology) and toward the tissue cell–specific model (intracrinology). The effects of prohormones at their target tissue sites rather than blood levels are now being thought of as the better measurement of hormonal activity.

What does this mean to the average patient? Intracrinology will enable a more accurate view of what is "really going on" at the cell level, resulting in a more complete and accurate understanding of human physiology. When mainstream endocrinology embraces the new generation of testosterone prohormones, advanced intracrinology research will follow.

KARLIS ULLIS, M.D.
Sports Medicine & Anti-Aging Medical Group
1807 Wilshire Blvd., Suite 205
Santa Monica, CA 94003
Phone: (310) 829-1990
Fax: (310) 829-5134
E-mail: kulllis@ucla.edu
Website:http://www.agingprevent.com

Introduction

Two watershed events occurred in 1998 that changed the public's perception of sexuality and supplements. The first was the introduction of Viagra, the little blue diamond-shaped pill that marked the first scientifically verified drug to reverse male impotency for up to 6 hours. The second was baseball's home run king Mark McGwire's record-breaking season.

What did the first have to do with the second? With all deference to Mark, his incredible skills at home plate were far less important from a medical standpoint than the publicity resulting from the revelation that he used androstenedione. Had an enterprising reporter not spotted a bottle of pills containing the little-known substance in Mark's locker room, it might have been years before the public was introduced to the most important breakthrough ever in naturally occurring sexual hormone-boosting supplements. The connection between the two substances has to do with the duality of human sexuality: desire and function. (Desire usually precedes sexual activity.) Viagra restored sexual prowess to men with erectile dysfunction. Essentially, it works by suppressing an enzyme that blocks the dilation of blood vessels inside the male and female genitalia. (Obviously, the results are more pronounced with men.) What it doesn't do is affect sexual desire—or, in Freudian terms, libido, a human trait found in no other animal.

For all other species, sex is a reflex, the biochemically induced means for procreation. When the female is in sexual heat, or estrous, the male reflexively mounts her. That defines the sexual experience in animals. For humans, sex is far more complex and only sometimes has to do with procreation. Coitus begins with a fantasy that evolves into increased sexual interest, which in turn increases motivation for sexual activity. Mix in the societal norms, religion, age, health, and gender, and sex becomes a many splendored but sometimes complicated thing.

The medical community and the public quickly discovered that Viagra worked only on the mechanical part of the human sexual equation and did nothing for desire. A man might now be able to obtain an erection, but did he want to have sex? And what about women's libido? Viagra does nothing for sexual desire because it only works to dilate blood vessels and has no direct effect on the brain.

Then came the 1998 baseball season. Mark McGwire's training regimen shed light on the new development of a group of substances called "testosterone prohormones"; androstenedione was only one of many. Actually, testosterone prohormones—or "T-boosters," as they've become known—were introduced in 1996, but the public barely took notice. It's ironic because they were immediately available as over-the-counter supplements at a fraction of the cost of Viagra. The difference in how Viagra and T-boosters were ushered into the public arena has everything to do with modern-day pharmaceutical medicine. Since Viagra is a synthetic drug, its manufacturer, Pfizer, could file a patent to prevent other companies from replicating its formula. T-boosters, on the other hand, are naturally occurring substances in the human body and in nature, and thus are not eligible for patents. A dozen companies or more now sell T-boosters over the counter in health food stores and drugstores and via the Internet.

So what do T-boosters have to do with making Mark McGwire a better home run slugger? The answer is testosterone. There is no other substance on the planet, natural or man-made, that can have such profound effects on human physiology. Testosterone has an almost mystical reputation as being responsible for all things aggressive and manly. But that is more of a popular misconception than it is science, for it is an essential hormone for women too, albeit in smaller amounts.

Testosterone can restore or boost sex drive in men and women, but it has numerous other health benefits, including decreasing fat tissue and increasing muscle mass. Its ability to make dramatic improvements in the human physique is why McGwire, bodybuilders, and probably many other professional athletes use it. It also can "sharpen the mind" and build confidence. Testosterone is necessary to complete the male and female sexual experience. It increases the overall energy levels needed by both sexes for the muscular and mental activity during lovemaking. Without an adequate supply of testosterone, a Viagra-aided sexual experience is unsatisfying.

Now, for the first time in history, anyone can walk into a health food store, buy a T-booster supplement, and within minutes have elevated levels of testosterone. In terms of biochemistry, T-boosters are "precursors" to testosterone, which means they are one step and one molecule removed from testosterone. A T-booster becomes testosterone by a single, simple chemical reaction. A T-booster gum may soon be available; its popularity among professional baseball players and weekend warriors can only be imagined.

As a medical doctor for more than twenty years who has worked with elite athletes in five Olympic Games, as well as hundreds of average men and women, I am conflicted over the easy availability of T-boosters. In my private practice at the Sports Medicine and Anti-Aging Medical Group in Santa Monica, California, I have prescribed testosterone for years as part of an overall regimen for both better sex, a better body, and more energy. The results have been dramatic. I have seen the lives of patients changed. Couples have had their sex lives restored. Baby boomers have delayed retirement because of the new burst of energy and confidence. On the other hand, testosterone is a powerful hormone. While in my clinical practice T-boosters have proven to have no or minimal undesirable side effects, one has only to observe the abuse of Viagra by sexually well functioning men to be concerned about the possible misuse of T-boosters.

The testosterone genie is out of the bottle, however. Dozens of different types of T-booster combinations are now available as over-the-counter products. To the uninformed, buying T-boosters can be confusing and potentially dangerous. I wrote this book to allow men and women to use these new wonder supplements in a safe and effective way. With the guidance provided in the following pages, you will be able make intelligent choices about their use in your own health and fitness regimen. This book is not intended for those wishing to boost their testosterone levels into the upper stratosphere. Rather, it's for all of us who want to avoid the maladies of middle age associated with a decline in testosterone, including increased incidence of diabetes, heart disease, depressed mood, and a decrease in cognitive abilities and, yes, sexual desire and performance.

In Part I of *Super T, Sex-Enhancing Supplements,* we review the myths and medical science of testosterone and T-boosters as well as other substances sold as sexual enhancers. Part II, The Natural Body Makeover, provides a personalized fat-loss and muscle-building program. Part III, Better Sex, discusses in depth the sexual component of testosterone and provides a supplement regimen designed to improve your love life and, if you're using Viagra, a way to maximize its effect. In Part IV, Your Personal T-Booster Regimen, we put it all together to create a regimen of supplements, diet, and exercise that is suited to your individual needs.

To use this book most effectively, first decide which of three major goals you would like to accomplish that can be assisted by T-boosters: fat loss, muscle gain, or sexual enhancement. Don't worry: These goals are not mutually exclusive, although each utilizes T-boosters in a slightly different way. By setting your priorities you can ensure safety and a minimum of duplication of effort. With your foundation program in place, you can then modify it to accomplish other goals. Chapter 9 provides a handy "day planner" for recording the various components of your T-booster regimen, while Chapter 10 provides a consumer's guide—complete with ratings—to popular pro-sexual supplements.

This is the dawning of a new sexual revolution. Hormones that just a few years ago were barely understood are now sold like candy. We must proceed with caution, but there is no turning back. This book will ensure that you won't be left behind in this era of powerful supplements—without putting your health at risk.

◦⊷ Part I ⊶◦

Sex-Enhancing
Supplements

·◄ 1 ►·

The Dawn of the
T-Booster Era

While I have been using natural testosterone therapies in my private practice for years, only recently has testosterone become part of mainstream medicine. Medical researchers have known for decades of the benefits of the hormone, but its powerful effects have scared many physicians. The fact that bodybuilders and athletes took matters into their own hands in the seventies and began using synthetic anabolic steroid drugs to boost testosterone levels further alienated the medical establishment from considering the benefits of testosterone therapies.

Then in 1994, despite much teeth gnashing from the American Medical Association and intense lobbying from the pharmaceutical industry, Congress enacted the Dietary, Supplement and Health Education Act. This groundbreaking legislation permitted the sale directly to the consumer of "natural" substances. If it was found in nature or the human body, the U.S. Government said it was legal to sell "over the counter," or without a prescription.

Although this landmark legislation may be news to you, you are probably familiar with its consequences. Melatonin and DHEA were among the first phase of products that were released under the new act. Now we are witnessing phase two: the release of testosterone prohormones, also known as T-boosters.

What is the power of T-boosters? Because they are almost identical in chemical structure to testosterone itself, they can alter the sexual hormone mix of the body. When used intelligently, T-boosters and their related biochemical kin can rekindle sexual drive. In fact, if you think that Viagra is the answer to all your sexual problems, by the time you've finished this book, you may conclude that T-boosters (which are available at a fraction of the cost of Viagra) are actually more effective.

If enhancing sexuality is not enough, T-boosters have the capacity to reverse the bane of almost all baby boomers—middle-aged spread. Taken properly, they can safely and effectively reduce fat and increase muscle mass in a way that no diet by itself can. Finally, T-boosters can energize like coffee but without the jittery effects of caffeine. They can also increase physical endurance, which, when combined with a pro-testosterone diet and exercise, can be an effective tool in an overall antiaging health and fitness regimen.

Make no mistake: T-boosters are powerful supplements and must be used carefully. Our first rule is easy to remember: Start Low and Go Slow. That means always start with the *lowest* possible dosage of T-boosters and use them as infrequently as possible until an effective level is reached. You will receive guidelines in the upcoming pages concerning the beginning of this process, but it's incumbent on you as a good student of sex hormone physiology to read and understand the information presented here—*especially* the precautions—before taking any T-booster or other hormonal supplement.

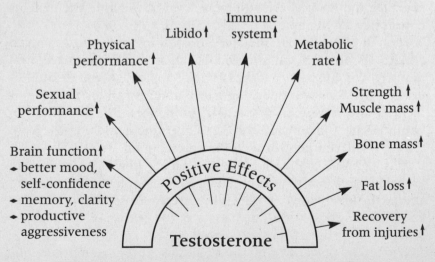

FIGURE 1—*Testosterone Effects in Adult Men and Women*

The Search for the Miracle Hormone

Testosterone enhances sexual desire while burning fat and increasing muscle. Is there any wonder that it has been considered "the miracle hormone"? Surprisingly, not until 1935 when it was first isolated were scientists even sure that the hormone existed, although it had been the subject of speculation for centuries. History records that in 1400 B.C. in India, testicular extracts from animals were recommended for improving sexual performance in men. In 1792 an English scientist named John Hunter tried removing the testicles from cocks and transplanting them to hens, but this crude experiment was not successful. The German proto-endocrinologist Arnold Adolph Berthold began similar research in 1848 by transplanting rooster testicles into castrated roosters and observing their behavior. Berthold claimed the testicles made the castrated roosters more active and aggressive.

About fifty years later a French scientist named Charles-Edouard Brown-Séquard injected himself with a crude blend of guinea pig and dog testes. He swore that it gave him an amazing boost of energy, increased his sex drive, and, in medical science's first pissing contest, even increased the arc of his urinary stream. Brown-Séquard was actually a very well respected doctor and medical researcher responsible for several notable medical discoveries, but nonetheless he soon became the laughingstock of the scientific world.

In the 1920s, the first organized and sustained research to find this sex hormone began under the auspices of Squibb Pharmaceuticals at the University of Chicago. Led by Fred C. Koch, this team risked the same ridicule that Brown-Séquard endured for his efforts. A mixture made from bull testicles was injected into castrated roosters daily for two weeks. Lo and behold, this mixture proved effective at restoring some of the castrated roosters' manhood. The study was repeated with the same result, and thus it became the first scientifically verifiable study documenting the effects of a male sex hormone.

Testosterone Discovered

Now the race was on to actually isolate the substance. A group of German scientists led by Adolf Butenandt was determined to find the male hormone. This involved a number of comical approaches, including the distillation of twenty-five thousand liters of policemen's urine and mashing up two thousand pounds of bull testicles. But these extraordinary methods finally paid off in 1935 when a group of Dutch scientists isolated testosterone from mice testes. Later that year the German research team successfully synthesized testosterone, winning Adolf Butenandt a Nobel Prize for his work.

Since 1935, testosterone's notoriety has increased tremendously. The Nazis during World War II were thought to have experimented with testosterone on soldiers of the Third Reich to make them more aggressive. Testosterone was tested in the 1940s for a wide variety of uses: to treat impotence, anemia, and low libido, and even to prevent muscle loss during dieting.

The first book on testosterone, entitled *The Male Hormone*, was published in 1945. This groundbreaking work was written by Paul de Kruif, a reporter with previous medical training. He described the prevailing unease that the medical community had with testosterone as "medical dynamite" and "sexual TNT." He argued that the strong sexual effects of testosterone on both men and women made many doctors nervous and prevented the medical community from taking the science of testosterone seriously. De Kruif himself was an avid testosterone user when he wrote:

> Now I'm fifty-four years old, and there's much left to do. I've grown old much too quickly. . . . Meanwhile I'll keep taking the methyl testosterone that now gives me the total vitality to go on working.

De Kruif was also one of the first to suggest testosterone as a performance enhancer for athletes:

> We know how both the St. Louis Cardinals and St. Louis Browns have won championships, super-charged by vitamins.

It would be interesting to watch the productive power of an industry or a professional group that would try a systematic supercharge with testosterone.

Advent of Anabolic Steroids

In 1956 a doctor named John Ziegler attended the World Games in Moscow and discovered that Russian athletes were using testosterone. Impressed by their success, he was determined to give American athletes the same advantage. His concerns over the many side effects of testosterone were alleviated when CIBA pharmaceuticals developed Dianabol, a synthetic drug closely related in its molecular structure to testosterone. Taken in pill form, Dianabol did produce rapid muscle gain in athletes and had fewer side effects than testosterone. Another advantage over testosterone was that it did not have to be injected. Word spread quickly among the athletic community, and soon Dianabol was nicknamed the "Breakfast of Champions."

Shortly after the development of Dianabol, pharmaceutical companies began to develop even more sophisticated derivatives of testosterone. A flood of new synthetic anabolic hormone steroids such as Deca Durabolin, Anavar, and Primabolan hit the medical market. These new drugs were studied for many medical uses, including treatment for underweight patients, for osteoporosis, for growth-deficient children, and for anemia. And as with Dianabol, the use of these new drugs spread rapidly among athletes.

Synthetic anabolic hormone steroids—or "steroids," as they would become known (somewhat inaccurately)—were used not only by Russian weight lifters but by every country's athletes and in every sport. The biggest users were weight lifters, track and field athletes, and football players. By one estimate, one-third of the U.S. track and field team used steroids in preparation for the 1968 Olympic Games in Mexico City.

By the late 1960s sports governing bodies succeeded in banning anabolic steroid use from most international sports competition. The one exception was the growing and unconventional sport of bodybuilding. Despite the official ban, a huge percentage of these Olympic and professional athletes were believed to use them regularly. Indeed, it is thought that many world records set in the early seventies that have yet to be broken were achieved with the influence of anabolic steroids.

In the 1970s many in the medical community sought to prove the toxicity and ineffectiveness of anabolic steroids. At the 1976 American College of Sports Medicine meeting, studies were presented that showed a lack of effect of anabolic steroids. Many of these studies were poorly designed and would later be discredited, but the prevailing mood in the medical community at this time was strongly "antisteroid."

Crude techniques for testing athletes for steroid use were first used in 1976, and some—but not all—steroid-using athletes were disqualified from international competition as a result. By 1983 extremely sensitive equipment for drug testing was developed, and when it was used for the first time in the Pan American Games in Caracas, Venezuela, many American athletes excused themselves from participating because of "family emergencies." By the Los Angeles 1984 Olympic Games, state-of-the-art gas chromatographic and mass spectroscopy equipment made steroid use much more difficult.

The most famous steroid case came in 1988 when Canadian runner Ben Johnson was stripped of his gold medal after testing positive for steroids. Ironically, many experts have argued that Johnson was more deserving of this medal than his competitors because the steroid he was using was actually very weak. It is likely that his competitors were using much stronger and more sophisticated steroids that would not show up in tests. One anonymous Soviet coach was quoted as saying, "I feel sorry for Ben Johnson. Ninety percent of all sportsmen, including our own, use steroid drugs."

The worldwide publicity over the Johnson incident fanned the flames of antisteroid hysteria. By this time a conservative estimate was that one million people used anabolic steroids in the United States. Several published medical studies recommended classification of anabolic steroids as controlled substances. Hearings held in the U.S. Senate in 1989 included compelling testimony from several professional and Olympic athletes describing the intense pressure to improve their performance by using anabolic steroids.

In 1990 the federal Steroid Trafficking Act was passed, which made it illegal to possess or sell steroids and imposed stricter regulations on its medical use. The prison terms for illegal possession and sale were close to those for cocaine possession and sale. Many pharmaceutical companies removed their brands from the market to avoid trouble with federal authorities. Several doctors were actually sent to prison for overprescribing anabolic steroids.

In spite of the stricter laws and bad publicity, research on testosterone continued. The HIV/AIDS crisis resulted in expanded use of anabolic steroids to prevent muscle wasting in sufferers, but it was not until 1996 that the most definitive and conclusive research study on testosterone was published.

Breakthrough Study

New research not only verified the extraordinary effectiveness of testosterone but also shows that it is far safer and has far fewer side effects than previously believed. In groundbreaking research in 1995, a group of scientists, led by Shalender Bhasin, M.D., professor and chairman of endocrinology at the UCLA Charles Drew School of Medicine, conducted an extremely bold medical study in which the effectiveness of testosterone was tested by giving large doses to normal healthy men between the ages of nineteen and forty. Over ten weeks, twenty-two men received weekly intramuscular injections of 600 milligrams of testosterone enenthate, a dose that causes testosterone levels to rise up to five times above normal (also known as "supraphysiological" levels). Another group of twenty-one men were given a placebo. Keep in mind that even for a male with very low testosterone levels, the average intramuscular replacement dose is 50 to 100 milligrams per week.

Most medical researchers predicted that the men receiving such high doses would experience numerous adverse psychological and medical side effects, including extreme aggression. Instead, the test subjects receiving testosterone did not experience any adverse mood disturbance and scored in the normal range on psychological tests rating mood and aggression. In fact, no abnormal behavior was observed whatsoever.

Two other preconceptions about testosterone were challenged by the Bhasin study. It was thought that high levels of testosterone would significantly lower good HDL-cholesterol levels and increase the risk of prostate cancer. In fact, the study revealed no statistically significant drop in these levels. It must be noted, though, that these men were on a very controlled low-fat diet. Also, there were no elevated PSA levels among the men to indicate prostate problems. On the other hand, the men taking testosterone did experience a 7 to 9 percent increase in lean fat-free mass. Even the men who did not exercise experienced more increase in muscle mass than men who exercised without testosterone.

The medical community could no longer claim that testosterone was a dangerous and ineffective hormone. If taking unnaturally high doses of synthetic testosterone proved to be safe, naturally raising testosterone levels within the normal range should pose no extraordinary health risks. This is not to say that a person should inject himself with massive doses of testosterone if he could gain access to it (it must be prescribed by a licensed physician). It is important to keep in mind that all the subjects in the study were prescreened for medical conditions and the testosterone was given under close medical supervision.

The Science of Testosterone

Bhasin's study made it acceptable for medical science to study testosterone again. Subsequent research has destroyed two other myths about the hormone: that it only affects sexuality and that it only affects men.

Testosterone affects men *and* women, and acts on various tissues, from the brain to bones and muscles. It varies in amount and pattern of secretion between the genders, but just as men must have some estrogen to function normally, women need testosterone throughout their lives for good health. Scientists have divided the actions of testosterone into two main categories: *androgenic* and *anabolic*. The androgenic effects of testosterone are known as masculinizing or virilizing. These include the growth of body and facial hair, male sex organ development (or the enlargement of the female clitoris), deepening of the voice, and male pattern baldness.

Testosterone by itself actually has relatively few androgenic effects, but it converts to another hormone known as dihydrotestosterone

(DHT), which is much more androgenic than testosterone. DHT causes many of the side effects that testosterone is blamed for, including acne, enlarged prostate, and male pattern baldness. Actually, only a small percentage of testosterone converts to DHT, but taken in excess, it can lead to high DHT levels and, thus, more side effects.

Testosterone is well known for its energizing effect and for increasing sexual interest in both men and women. It also can increase a person's confidence level and may express itself as aggressiveness in persons who are not mentally balanced. I have seen huge changes in the personalities of men and women with depressed testosterone levels; they become happy, confident, and energized people when their testosterone levels are returned to a normal range.

One of the reasons for testosterone's popularity among athletes is the immediacy of its effects. Taken before exercising, it can result in dramatic improvements in performance, partly through its direct brain-stimulating properties, which occurs within minutes.

The other significant aspect of testosterone's activity is its anabolic effects. Anabolic refers to testosterone's powerful capacity to stimulate the growth of muscle, bone, and red blood cells. The growth of muscle is useful not only for athletes but for anyone seeking a better body. The anabolic effect on bones and red blood cells has also led to the use of testosterone for osteoporosis (excess loss of bone) and anemia (low red blood cell levels).

Testosterone's effects on sex drive, fat loss, and muscle mass gain are the areas where it can make the biggest difference in people's lives.

New Era of T-Boosters

In 1996 a brilliant young chemist named Patrick Arnold came up with the idea of making and selling natural, over-the-counter testosterone boosters. Arnold had experience working as an industrial chemist but found the work dull and soon decided to use his talent and expertise for his true passion—bodybuilding. After a brief stint at a major sports nutrition company, Arnold decided he could be more successful as an independent supplement developer and teamed up with a chemical manufacturer to develop the first over-the-counter formula containing the previously obscure testosterone pro-hormone androstenedione, a naturally occurring substance that your body uses to make testosterone. Androstenedione, or just adione, had previously been used as part of the East German Olympic team's steroid program, but American athletes and sports nutrition companies had not paid much attention to it. Shortly after the introduction of androstenedione, Arnold began to sell and manufacture an even more obscure, natural hormone called 4-androstenediol, also known as 4-adiol. New research confirmed previous studies that 4-androstenediol can boost testosterone even more than androstenedione.

Androstenedione and 4-androstenediol work in similar ways. Both are hormones extremely close in structure to testosterone. Once they are ingested, the body naturally converts these hormones into testosterone through the action of different enzymes. The advantage to taking these new supplements rather than testosterone is that the body has a limited capacity to convert 4-androstenediol and androstenedione to testosterone, so these products will boost testosterone but only to normal and natural levels permitted by the body.

Today, T-boosters compete in a dynamic consumer marketplace of sexual supplements. The shelves of a typical health food store are overflowing with products that claim to increase sexual drive and enhance performance. For the consumer this new era is exciting in terms of its immediate accessibility and comparative affordability, but for a physician it is worrisome in its potential for abuse. In the next two chapters we will separate the safe and effective products from the bad and bogus.

- 2 -

The First Generation of Sex Enhancers

The development and sale of T-boosters in 1996 marked a dividing line between the new generation of sexually enhancing T-boosters and the old generation of pills, potions, herbs, and snake oil that claimed to be aphrodisiacs.

T-booster prohormones promote the elevation of testosterone in the blood and tissues and can alter the testosterone-to-estrogen ratios. Chapters 7 and 8 will explain how the ratio between the male and female hormones has a powerful effect on sexual, general physical, and mental health. To a comparatively large degree we can control and influence the effects of the new generation T-boosters.

The older generation of sex enhancers were crude in their approach and unpredictable in their results, but they were the culmination of mankind's single-minded search for ways to enhance sexual prowess for thousands of years. Many of the love potions and aphrodisiacs used throughout history may seem comical or in some cases repugnant, but they merely illustrate the strong motivation to find effective sex boosters.

One legendary way of enhancing sex has been through eating animal genitalia. The practice of eating animal parts is known as *organotherapy* and was extremely popular during the height of the Roman Empire. Just as it was thought that eating animals' hearts would boost courage, it was also believed that eating penises, wombs, and testes from almost any animal would enhance human sexuality.

Theoretically, one could derive a small boost in testosterone, and thus enhance sex drive, by eating large quantities of animal organs containing testosterone. More likely the supposed effect was psychological.

Another legendary aphrodisiac is Spanish fly, a powder consisting of ground parts of a beetle known as *Cantharis vesicatoria*. It has been in use since antiquity and was mentioned by Hippocrates. The Roman empress Livia was said to have slipped Spanish fly into the food of her rivals to induce improper sexual behavior that she could use against them. Actually, Spanish fly can be toxic, and its supposed libido-enhancing effects are merely a myth. Use of Spanish fly, however, can lead to itching and irritation in the genitals.

Roman women highly valued the sweat of gladiators. Soap was not invented until the Middle Ages, so the Romans cleansed themselves with olive oil, applying it like suntan lotion and then gently scraping it off. This appetizing combination of male perspiration and olive oil was thought to drive women wild when ingested, and the more macho the man, the more powerful the effect. Champion gladiators bottled their used bath "soap" and derived a substantial income from their sweat—without the toil.

The quest to find the magic bullet for boosting sexual interest and sexual activity, and improving performance, continues. You will find at your local health food store or drugstore a wide variety of formulas that supposedly will give your sex life a boost. You should be careful what you buy, however. Some of these supplements are based on science, at least on a rudimentary level, while others are based on myth and legend. In general, these formulas have not proven to be effective.

When Viagra became available in March 1998, it rang up an estimated $1 billion in sales by the end of the year. Considering what else was available, there should be little surprise at its meteoric success. The pharmaceutical industry is now rushing to find more products for this market, including female sexual enhancers. Previously, the industry had entirely ignored the development of products for women's sexual needs. As one might expect, less than scrupulous supplement manufacturers are jumping on the gravy train and rolling out products touted as complementary to Viagra, and there are even female versions of Viagra (whatever that means). However, while all the new agents are for boosting performance, most of them fail to address the primary and fundamental aspect of human sexuality known clinically as "sexual interest." What good is the ability to perform if there is no interest in sex?

In this sense, the first generation of sexual-enhancing substances was not totally without merit. Many of these products may also help boost the effectiveness of Viagra and T-boosters even if they have only a mild effect on their own. Other supplements sold as sex boosters may not be effective at increasing libido or erections but may have many other health benefits.

In this chapter we'll wrestle with the good, the bad, and the ugly of the first generation of sexual enhancers: from basic minerals and exotic herbs to the newer quasi-amino acid supplements such as acetyl L-carnitine and the hormone DHEA. When the dust settles, we'll have a pretty good idea as to what, besides T-boosters and Viagra, is worth considering.

Minerals

Minerals are essential elements for proper body function. Certain minerals are needed in your diet for proper hormone production and, ergo, a healthy sex life. Numerous supplement manufacturers have marketed minerals over the last decade as a direct means of boosting testosterone. Research and my own clinical experience indicate that only one mineral has an effect on testosterone: zinc.

Zinc

This mineral is essential for good health and specifically for testosterone production. It probably influences the action of the enzymes that lead to testosterone synthesis from prohormones (including adione and adiol). While the exact role of zinc in testosterone production has not been determined, low levels of zinc have been linked to low testosterone levels, poor prostate function, and decreased sperm count. One study showed that zinc deficiency led to more testosterone being converted to estrogen. Another study showed that impotent men were more likely to have low levels of zinc, possibly due to their low testosterone levels.

Oysters are high in zinc, and this is perhaps the reason why oysters have a reputation as an aphrodisiac. However, if you are getting enough zinc in your diet, taking extra zinc will not increase your testosterone production. Many supplement companies sell zinc as a testosterone-boosting formula, but don't expect huge results unless you have a poor diet and are zinc deficient.

Some companies sell zinc lozenges as a treatment for the common cold. Zinc is essential for proper immune function and has a link to antiviral systems of the body, but be careful not to take too *much* zinc. Large doses of zinc will not improve immunity and may actually *decrease* immunity. In addition, large doses of zinc can interfere with absorption of other essential minerals. To be safe, keep your doses of zinc to no more than 50 milligrams while you are sick. When not sick, keep zinc consumption to 15 to 25 milligrams a day.

Boron

This mineral has been advertised on the back pages of many body-building magazines as a "legal steroid alternative." The source of this claim is a single study that showed boron supplementation increased testosterone levels in postmenopausal women. It doesn't take a research scientist to know, however, that what works on postmenopausal women will not necessarily work in the rest of the population. Men and premenopausal women will likely not notice any effect from taking boron, but it may help to make the bones of postmenopausal women stronger by enhancing their estrogen levels.

This is not to say that boron is worthless as a supplement. It is an essential nutrient, so it's a good idea to take 3 milligrams of boron per day as part of a daily multimineral supplementation. In addition, boron is essential for bone health, and is an especially important supplement for those at risk for osteoporosis. Some research also shows that boron provides chemicals called hydroxyl groups, which are essential for the production of some steroid hormones. Be aware, though, that taking excess boron will not increase testosterone levels despite all the hype.

Food Extracts

Oysters

Oysters have long been considered a natural libido booster. The legendary lover Casanova was said to have eaten fifty raw oysters a day to help him keep up with his numerous sexual conquests. In the seventeenth-century Netherlands, oysters gained a strong reputation as a potent sexual enhancer.

As previously mentioned, oysters are high in zinc, which is essential for testosterone synthesis. However, it is much cheaper to take a multimineral supplement that includes zinc than to buy an expensive oyster extract supplement.

Oysters also contain tyrosine, an amino acid that may boost libido by stimulating the production of dopamine, a brain chemical messenger linked to sexual arousal and pleasure. Again, it is more cost effective to simply buy a tyrosine supplement. You can also eat almost any protein food to obtain tyrosine. L-tyrosine capsules at doses of 100 to 500 milligrams on an empty stomach can potentially act as a sexual stimulant by increasing your level of alertness and arousal through increasing the production of dopamine in the brain.

Orchic Extract

This is simply a polite term for "testicle extract," which could be from bulls or other animals, including horses, sheep, and goats. It is true that bull testicles contain testosterone and other hormones, but the amounts in most orchic extract supplements are minuscule and will not be well absorbed anyway. Gonadal glandular extracts could have some effect on persons who are very sensitive or are very depleted of hormones.

Eating animal gonads not only is unappealing to most of us but also poses a risk. Organ meats are breeding grounds for bacterial, viral, and other infectious diseases, including "mad cow disease." Nevertheless, in Europe, Mexico, and Asia, testicle extract or "live cell" injections are available and are even popular with some very wealthy but naive "potency seekers."

Other animal products include velvet deer horn extracts and Siberian deer horn extracts (also known as Pantocrine and Kantorine in Russia). Salmon eggs in Norway are called Libido. All of these substances contain a multitude of ingredients that are very hard to identify, and their effects are weak and unpredictable. Save your money and avoid orchic extract supplements altogether.

Herbs

The healing properties of certain herbs is undisputed. Medicinal herbs have been employed for centuries in almost every culture to prevent and cure various ailments. What is less certain is how herbal extracts affect sexual activity. Some herbs appear to counteract sexual inhibition. In this sense, herbs such as damiana are aphrodisiacs in the same way as alcohol. (As Ogden Nash once quipped, "Candy is dandy, but liquor is quicker.") Other herbs, such as gingko biloba, mimic the actions of Viagra (or is it the other way around?) and enhance sexuality by increasing blood flow to the sexual organs. Still others, such as saw palmetto, reduce irritation to male genitalia that might interfere in sexual enjoyment.

For our purposes, the most interesting herbs are those that may actually convert to testosterone. There is research that indicates both sarsaparilla and Avena sativa (green oats) may cause testosterone levels to rise gradually over a long period, that is, a month or more. In comparison, T-boosters take usually less than an hour.

Ginseng

Ginseng has been used in China for five thousand years as a tonic to heal, revitalize, and help adapt the human body to harsh environments. Its genus name, *Panax*, is derived from Greek words meaning "heal all." Panax ginseng is considered an adaptogenic type of herb, which means that it helps the body adapt to physical stress; specifically, it is believed to help improve physical stamina as well as enhance immune function. Ginseng has a long reputation for being a potent energizer and sexual enhancer. Studies show that it does have a mild stimulant effect, and some men have noticed improved sexual performance after taking ginseng.

The exact mechanism by which ginseng improves sexual function is not known, but ginseng likely increases sexuality indirectly by giving men and women greater energy and an overall higher alertness level. It may also decrease depressive symptoms and the attendant affects of physical inertia and low sexual interest. Coffee works similarly, and studies have shown that coffee drinkers on the average have more sex than those who abstain. They also have lower suicide rates, so both effects are probably the result of the dopamine and catecholamine neurotransmitter systems that increase the release of epinephrine, dopamine, and norepinephrine. Too much release of the catecholamines, adrenaline-like substances, may lead to increased anxiety, especially in men who are already anxious and have psychological erectile dysfunction.

The potency of ginseng varies tremendously. You may have to try several different brands and types of ginseng before you notice any effect. If you really feel that ginseng is for you or want to experiment with it, then be sure to buy your ginseng from a reputable source known for selling truly potent ginseng. Avoid buying canned or preserved ginseng.

Oddly enough, most of the Chinese I have spoken to in my travels throughout Asia prefer the "cool American Wild Wisconsin" ginseng. Slice the root thinly and then cook overnight in an electric cooking pot. Then drink and eat the soft root as needed. Ginseng should not be used for more than two to four weeks at a time.

•→ *Caution:* Don't use ginseng if you have high blood pressure or are "stimulant sensitive."

Ginkgo biloba

The ginkgo biloba tree is the oldest surviving tree species. The tree was first discovered in ancient China, where the emperor Shen Nung hailed ginkgo as "good for the heart and lungs." The trees were planted in Japan about one thousand years ago, and now they grow throughout the world, including the United States.

Ginkgo works mainly through the unique glycoside compounds found in the leaf. Ginkgo effects include antioxidant and anti-inflammatory properties, decreasing stickiness of platelets (a blood thinning effect like aspirin), increased brain cell activity for neurotransmitter communication signals, increased glucose use by the brain (giving it more energy), and overall improvement and regulation of blood flow throughout the brain and body. In Europe it is often prescribed by doctors as a memory booster and treatment for Alzheimer's disease.

A 1989 study shows that ginkgo has promise in treating impotence. Sixty patients with erectile dysfunction who had failed to respond to previous treatments were given 60 milligrams a day of ginkgo biloba extract for six months. An impressive 50 percent were able to have better erections after six months, with 25 percent experiencing improved blood flow in the arteries.

Gingko may be a good pro-sexual adjunct to T-boosters for those whose lifestyles or diseases have led them to have poor blood flow— such as smokers and those with arterial narrowing, diabetes, high lipid blood levels (high cholesterol), and so on. For that matter, alpha lipoic acid, magnesium, acetyl L-carnitine, vitamin E, and other agents can help with overall poor blood flow in the small blood vessels as well as increase insulin action and cell sensitivity to insulin. That is important because the three major causes of low testosterone levels and erectile dysfunction in men are cardiac disease, smoking, and diabetes.

•→ *Caution:* This powerful herb should be used with caution or not used at all in patients on aspirin or Coumadin or other therapies for thinning the blood, or who have uncontrolled hypertension, bleeding problems, or prior hemorrhagic strokes. Its use should be stopped for some weeks before surgery. You should always consult with your doctor concerning your clotting capacity if you have any bleeding risk factors.

Saw Palmetto

The saw palmetto plant (*Serenoa repens*) is a species of dwarf palm tree that grows in the southeastern United States, especially in Florida. The crushed berries from these plants were consumed for centuries by various Native American tribes. They believed that saw palmetto had good nutritional benefits and was good for genital and reproductive health.

The berry contains three main compounds, including plant

sterols, a steroid-like structure. For this reason it has been sold as a "plant steroid" or as a "steroid replacement" or "sex-enhancing" supplement. However, it may have the opposite effect. This is the main reason it has been used by men to decrease the effects of the testosterone metabolic product called dihydrotestosterone (DHT), which is abundantly found in the prostate gland. One study showed that saw palmetto actually blocks testosterone receptors.

Saw palmetto may have a mild stimulatory effect and could motivate one to engage in sexual activity. These effects are probably secondary to improvement of prostate and urinary function. There is no evidence that saw palmetto has any positive effect on libido or muscle gain. Men with urinary difficulties, prostate inflammation, or an enlarged prostate may want to try saw palmetto as an alternative to prescription prostate medications. I recommend products that contain saw palmetto for prostate protection for male patients over forty with prostate problems who want to use T-boosters.

Pygeum

This herb (*Pygeum africanum*) comes from the bark extracts of a tropical evergreen tree grown in southern Africa. Several African tribes have used the herbal extracts from this tree as a tonic for urinary and genital health. Like saw palmetto, it contains substances with sterol structures and other compounds. One of these sterol compounds is called beta-sitosterol, which has also been sold as a "steroid alternative."

Pygeum, like saw palmetto, has been shown to improve sexual behavior by improving urinary function and decreasing prostate pain. There is no evidence, however, that it will improve libido or muscle gain. Take pygeum if you are concerned about urinary-prostate problems, but do not expect any noticeable testosterone-like effects.

Damiana

This is a small shrub (*Turnera aphrodisiaca*) with fragrant leaves that is grown throughout Latin America. The ancient Mayan civilization used it as a tonic for "giddiness and loss of balance" and as an aphrodisiac. As you can tell by its botanical name, it has a reputation as a libido enhancer. In fact, this supplement is now being marketed as the "female Viagra."

Damiana contains beta-sitosterol, which may account for some of its effects. In addition it contains several other compounds that may produce a mild stimulatory effect. Some herbalists recommend its use as an antidepressant, a headache treatment, and a laxative. It is logical to assume that a person who feels less depressed will have more sexual interest, but there are no clinical studies to support damiana's use as a sexual enhancer.

Sarsaparilla

A large woody vine that grows throughout Mexico, South America, and the Caribbean, sarsaparilla (*Smilax sarsaparilla*) has been used for centuries by native tribes as a general health tonic as well as a cure for sexual impotence. It was later discovered by European traders and developed a reputation as a cure for syphilis and other sexually transmitted diseases in Europe. It was even listed as a syphilis treatment in the first medical encyclopedia published in America, *U.S. Pharmacopoeia*. A 1942 study in the *New England Journal of Medicine* showed sarsaparilla to be an effective treatment for psoriasis (a skin disorder).

The herb has been promoted and sold as a bodybuilding supplement that supposedly boosts testosterone levels. The sexual and anabolic confusion arises because one of the molecules in the plant root is called "sarsapagenin," a plant saponin (a steroid-like chemical structure). The extract can be synthetically converted into testosterone in a laboratory. This reaction, however, does *not* take place when the extract is ingested.

Muira Puama

Also known as "potency wood," muira puama (*Ptychopetalum olacoides*) is a bush or a small tree found in the Brazilian Amazon region. The root and bark of this plant have been used for centuries by indigenous tribes for sexual impotence and many other purposes, including paralysis, rheumatism, weakness, and dysentery, and as a nervous system tonic. It was brought back by explorers to Europe, where it became a part of herbal medicine and a popular treatment for impotency.

Muira puama has recently gained a following as a sex enhancer for men. This is partly due to a study in France by Dr. Jacques Waynberg in 1990 in which muira puama extract was given to 262 men suffering from loss of libido or erectile dysfunction. Waynberg reported that 62 percent of men with loss of libido reported "a dynamic effect" with some improvement, and 51 percent with erection problems reported improvement.

Since this study did not have a control group, however, there is no way of telling if the effects were from muira puama or from a placebo effect. A study using both a placebo group and a group receiving the extract needs to be done before this herb can be accepted as a legitimate sex enhancer. Keep in mind that both libido and erectile function can be highly influenced by psychological factors, so the belief that you are taking a strong sex booster can cause you to have positive effects even if you are only taking a placebo.

Like damiana and sarsaparilla, muira puama contains beta-sitosterol, but its active ingredients may contain other stimulants that work in different ways. Anecdotal reports on this supplement have generally been more positive than for damiana and sarsaparilla.

Yohimbine

This herb (*Pausinystalia yohimbe*) contains an alpha-1 adrenergic receptor blocker chemical that is derived from the bark of an African yohimbé tree. Alpha adrenergic receptors are docking sites for chemical messengers that signal blood vessels to either relax or constrict. The penile blood vessels contain both alpha-1 and alpha-2 receptor-docking sites. When these sites are blocked, an influx of blood occurs that can result in erections. The opposite can occur when too much adrenaline is released, such as during anxiety, and the receptors are overstimulated.

Yohimbine bark extracts are often sold as a natural testosterone booster and libido enhancer. While it doesn't have any effect on testosterone levels, it is still a potent agent. It is also sold as a prescription medication for erectile dysfunction under the brand name Yocon as well as the generic name yohimbine hydrochloride. It was once sold as part of a prescription formula called Afrodex that contained yohimbine, strychnine, and testosterone. Afrodex was effective but controversial, and was pulled from the market by the FDA in 1973 due to safety concerns. Yohimbine is still available by prescription or as a bark extract supplement.

In addition to helping men obtain an erection, yohimbine may also boost libido. Sexual interest may increase because of its general nervous system stimulation effects. A 1984 study showed this effect on rats.

How does yohimbine extracts or prescription yohimbine compare to Viagra for improving erections? It is considerably weaker and more unpredictable, with many more undesirable side effects. Several studies on impotent men have shown a moderate level of effectiveness. In five separate studies, yohimbine has produced a positive response rate of 33 to 46 percent. This is much less than the 70 percent or more positive response rates reported in studies on Viagra.

Several studies have shown yohimbine to be moderately effective for increasing metabolism and mobilizing the use of fat for fuel. Fitness guru Dan Duchaine has also speculated that yohimbine may help mobilize fat in the lower bodies of women, a traditional "tough spot" for women trying to lose fat. A commercial yohimbine cream is sold to help reduce lower body fat, but its effectiveness has yet to be proven. Yohimbine is also sold as part of various "thermogenic" formulas designed to speed up the metabolism and decrease appetite.

•➤ *Caution:* Yohimbine has actions similar to those of Viagra and should not be taken at the same time. A synergistic action could produce a condition of painfully prolonged erections called priapism, a medical emergency that can result in permanent damage if left untreated. Do not take yohimbine if you are anxious or stressed, or have high blood pressure or a thyroid problem. Other possible side effects include sweating, nausea, headache, skin flushing, panic, and hallucinations.

Kava Kava

This Polynesian herb (*Piper methysticum*) has been used for centuries as a natural sedative and relaxant. It has recently gained popularity in the United States as a natural alternative to Valium and other tranquilizers. Kava kava does have a good record for being a mild relaxant, but its claim of enhanced libido in women is more suspect. No scientific studies have been conducted on the sexual aspect of kava kava. Some of my female patients have reported better sexual function with the use of kava kava as a mild relaxing and disinhibiting agent, an effect similar to that acquired by having a glass or two of wine or a small dose of a tranquilizer. In my clinical experience, I have not observed any effect of kava kava on sexual interest.

Avena Sativa (Green Oats)

Historically, the word "oats" has been associated with strength and sexuality. Expressions such as "sowing your wild oats" have become synonymous with masculinity and sexuality. In the eighteenth century oats were listed in the German pharmacopoeia as a sexual stimulant. An extract from a special breed of oats called *Avena sativa*— also known as "green oats" or "green oat straw"—has recently been widely sold both as a libido enhancer and as a testosterone booster.

The source of these claims comes from studies done at a graduate school in San Francisco called the Institute for Advanced Study of Human Sexuality. In one study, Avena sativa extracts were given to three men and three women for one month. Free testosterone (the active testosterone in the body) was measured at the beginning and end of the study. After one month, none of the women and one of the men had a change in free testosterone levels. However, two of the men had increased levels, one of 50 percent and the other of 185 percent.

While these increases are impressive, remember that there were only six people in the study, only two-thirds had changes in the free testosterone levels, and there was no placebo group in the study. A pill that supposedly increases libido and testosterone could cause a person to have various lifestyle changes (such as increased sex and exercise) that would raise testosterone levels in one month. Even the time of day that the blood samples were taken could influence free testosterone levels. More credible research needs to be conducted before any definitive conclusions can be reached.

In my own clinical experience, I have not observed elevations of free testosterone when patients were given Avena sativa extracts or products.

Stinging Nettle

Extracts from this plant (*Urtica dioica*) are often included in "male health" formulas with saw palmetto and pygeum. It has a reputation

as a libido enhancer and testosterone booster and also assists in urinary flow problems associated with enlarged prostate glands. These
effects have yet to be proven, although it has been widely researched
as a treatment for prostate enlargement throughout Europe and recently received some attention from American researchers.

Two German studies indicate that nettle may have some potential as a free testosterone booster. In this study, nettle extract was
shown to inhibit a blood protein called sex hormone binding globulin (SHBG), which has a high affinity for binding with testosterone.
When testosterone is "tied up or bound" to this specific protein, less
of the bioactive or free testosterone is around to do its normal job.
Thus, by decreasing SHBG, nettle may be able to increase free testosterone levels. However, this study was conducted *in vitro* (in a test
tube), so it is not clear if orally ingested nettle extract would have
the same effect in the live human body.

Most of the other studies on this herb showed beneficial effects
on the prostate and assisted urination with less residual urine in the
bladder, increased urinary flow, and decreased urinary frequency.

Amino Acids

Amino acids are essential substances like minerals that the body
needs in order to function properly. These nitrogen-containing, car-
bon-based compounds are of particular interest to bodybuilders
since they are a basic building block of protein from which muscle
is made. The more amino acids are delivered to the muscles, the
faster the muscular development.

In terms of sexuality, some amino acids have both a psychological
and a physiological function, enhancing libido, mood, and energy as
well as increasing blood flow. But their effects are indirect, and contrary to some advertisements, none are proven testosterone boosters.

L-tyrosine

This amino acid increases brain levels of the important brain messenger dopamine, which is essential for libido and energy. L-tyrosine is converted to L-dopa in the brain, which in turn makes
dopamine and then norepinephrine. All these substances are stim-

ulating and can increase sexual interest. If you are having problems with fatigue and low libido, try taking 100 to 500 milligrams of tyrosine on an empty stomach.

Caution: Use of L-tyrosine could result in the stimulation of growth of preexisting melanomas. Persons with skin pigmentation problems should consult a dermatologist before using these amino acids on an ongoing basis. They can also cause elevated blood pressure and excitement, and should not be used during pregnancy. Alternative whole food sources of tyrosine and phenylalanine include fish, turkey, chicken, milk products, and soy.

L-phenylalanine

Like tyrosine, this amino acid also increases dopamine levels and is a precursor to the manufacture of tyrosine. Some people get a better effect from tryosine, others from phenylalanine. Take 100 to 500 milligrams on an empty stomach for increased dopamine levels and a possible burst of energy, better mood, and enhanced sexual interest. Another form of phenylalanine, called DL-phenylalanine, has been sold as a natural pain reliever.

L-arginine

This amino acid is a natural source of nitrous oxide (NO), which is instrumental in the relaxation of blood vessels necessary in increasing blood flow to the penis for an erection. Prescription drugs such as phentolamine and prostaglandin E1 also increase NO, but unfortunately they need to be injected into the base of the penis to have any effect. Arginine can increase NO in the body when taken orally. Little scientific research has been done on its effects on erections, but it does show some promise.

Arginine may also improve fertility. One study showed arginine doubled sperm count in two weeks. For this reason it is given to male livestock animals if they are used as breeding stock.

Try taking .5 to 2 grams of arginine two or three times daily on an empty stomach if you are having erection or fertility problems. As an added bonus, arginine may also improve immunity. However, if

you have any form of herpes, you may want to avoid arginine because it can make herpes outbreaks worse. See chapter 7 on sexual
cocktails using L-arginine. Whole food sources of arginine are brazil
nuts, almonds, peanuts, lentils, kidney beans, soybeans, and sunflower seeds.

Acetyl L-carnitine (ALC)

This quasi-amino acid is sold by several sports nutrition companies
as a natural testosterone booster. The source of this claim is from one
study in rats, which is not necessarily applicable to humans. In addition, this study didn't show that ALC increased testosterone but,
rather, that it can prevent the drop in testosterone that occasionally
accompanies stress and overtraining.

ALC may be a helpful supplement to take before working out to
prevent testosterone from dropping and other symptoms of overtraining, but do not expect a big increase in testosterone. It has also
been studied extensively as a "smart drug" for improving memory
and concentration, and it is sold in Europe as a treatment for
Alzheimer's disease and other cognitive disorders.

Normal healthy people have also reported improvements in
mood, memory, and energy from taking ALC. Any substance that
enhances the sense of well-being and wellness is pro-sexual. Well-
being and health are highly associated with increased testosterone
levels and increased sexual interest and behavior. Overall, ALC has
many health benefits, but it is not a proven testosterone booster.

My clinical impression is that ALC improves neurologic function
and neurotransmission, and protects the energy factories in our cells
called the mitochondria. When the cells' and body's ability to generate energy are raised, the levels of sexuality and muscle building
capacity are raised as well.

Hormonal Compounds

Until the development and release of T-boosters in 1996, the closest
thing to genuine testosterone enhancers were two hormonal compounds, DHEA and pregnenolone. Both have varying positive effects, but their capacity to increase sexual drive is questionable.

DHEA

All the substances discussed so far may or may not enhance sexual drive, but none have proven capable of elevating testosterone levels. DHEA is different. Call it the first generation of T-boosters because it can, in fact, raise testosterone levels. The problem is that it can also have an opposite effect by raising estrogen levels, and there's no good way of knowing which will happen. It's the Russian roulette of anabolic hormones.

DHEA is the most abundant steroid hormone in the body. (A steroid molecular structure refers to the type of arrangement of four rings of carbon chains stuck together. Steroids in our body include cholesterol, pregnenolone, DHEA, progesterone, cortisol, estradiol, testosterone, androstenedione, androstenediol, and others.) DHEA is produced in our adrenal glands, the brain, and the skin. It has been widely researched and is the only supplement in this chapter that has been proven scientifically to raise testosterone levels.

DHEA was sold as an over-the-counter supplement during the early 1980s, but supplement companies were ordered to stop selling it in 1985. Many companies sold in its place wild yam extracts, which supposedly contained "natural DHEA." Actually, these supplements contain a compound similar to DHEA that can be converted into DHEA and other hormones only in the laboratory. In fact, some DHEA supplements, as well as the first birth control pills (containing estrogen and progesterone), are chemically synthesized from wild yam extracts. However, the human body lacks the enzymes to covert yam extracts into DHEA. Yam extracts have other health benefits, but they definitely are not a substitute for DHEA.

The Dietary Supplement Health and Education Act was passed in 1994, and real DHEA reappeared on the supplement market.

First isolated by scientists in 1934, DHEA can be converted to testosterone or estrogen in the human body, but only through a long process involving two separate chemical reactions and two different enzymes. Only a very small fraction of the original compound will end up as testosterone or estrogen. DHEA has not been shown to be a particularly strong testosterone booster or libido enhancer, but it may have many other health benefits. Much of its reputation is due to a 1994 study conducted at the University of California, San Diego, School of Medicine. Thirty male and female subjects aged forty to seventy were randomly assigned a placebo or 50 milligrams of DHEA to be taken daily for three months. The results of the study were impressive. The authors of the study stated that "DHEA supplementation resulted in a remarkable increase in perceived physical and psychological well-being for both men and women. The subjects reported increased energy, deeper sleep, improved mood, more relaxed feelings, and an improved ability to deal with stressful situations." However, *no* changes in libido were noticed by those taking DHEA in this study.

The San Diego medical researchers performed a follow-up study using double the dose of DHEA (100 milligrams a day) for twice the amount of time (six months). This study showed a strong increase in testosterone levels in both men and women, but unfortunately it did not measure the effects on libido. It did, however, show positive effects similar to the first study as well as increases in muscle mass.

While the effects of DHEA on libido are not definitive, the scientific research indicates that it is a moderately potent testosterone booster for women and only a mild one for men. It may therefore be a good choice for women seeking to increase their sex drive and is probably effective in men with extremely low sex hormone levels.

Caution: Women should be cautious when using it due to its high potency. Too much DHEA may cause a woman to grow facial hair and suffer from acne. Since it can also increase estrogen levels, women at risk for breast cancer should be especially cautious.

My clinical experience is that women derive greater benefits overall from DHEA than do men. My older or postmenopausal female patients have more energy, stronger bones, and better well-being after using DHEA with no serious side effects. The men in my clinic generally complain of a lack of sexual effect from DHEA; they mainly report a better sense of well-being and energy. Some of my middle-aged men even reported a *lowered* sexual interest; when I measured their hormones, I found that most of them had increased estrogen and lowered testosterone levels. (Their sexual desire returned a few weeks after abstaining from DHEA.) Overall, my younger male patients, twenty-five to thirty-five years of age, received the most positive effects from DHEA, perhaps because at that age they make less estrogen anyway. In general, men wishing to boost libido and testosterone levels would do better considering the new generation of T-boosters.

Despite being only a mildly effective T-booster, DHEA has many other health benefits, and some of the research on it looks promising. It has been studied for its positive effects on memory, immunity, lupus, cancer, heart disease, and many other problems. Its effects are not as great as much of the hype may lead you to believe, but if your DHEA levels have started to decline with age, you may wish to supplement it with small doses. If you are under forty years old, you probably have normal DHEA levels and will not benefit greatly from DHEA supplementation.

Pregnenolone

One other hormonal compound now sold as a supplement deserves mention. Pregnenolone is also an adrenal prohormone and like DHEA is a precursor to testosterone. It has been called "the mother hormone" since it is the second steroid hormone in the chain that starts with cholesterol. From it you can make many different hormones, including progesterone, DHEA, testosterone, estrogen, and cortisiol.

Pregnenolone helps some people feel more alert and have sharper memories. While pregnenolone is an important weapon in an anti-aging arsenal, overall it is not a "sexy" prohormone because one of its first conversion steps is to progesterone, which can be used to decrease sexual desire and behavior. Like DHEA, its effect on sexuality, if any, is unpredictable and most often may dampen sexuality in doses greater than 10 milligrams.

Take It Home

How do the first generation of sexual enhancers fit into modern pharmacology? At best they play a supporting role by either providing proper nutrients for overall good health or by eliminating problems that might inhibit sexual function, drive, and enjoyment. At worst they are a waste of money and potentially dangerous.

Two years ago, these substances were all we had. Today, as we'll explore in the next chapter, anyone can enjoy the benefit of a whole new generation of safe, effective, and fast-acting supplements that have taken the guesswork out of sexual enhancement.

.. 3 ..

The New Generation of T-Boosters and Sex Enhancers

The development and release in 1997 of T-boosters, a new type of over-the-counter supplement that can safely, effectively, and economically enhance testosterone levels, ushered in a new era in prosexual products. Previously, consumers wishing to increase their testosterone levels to achieve leaner bodies and better sex had to rely on relatively weak and often ineffectual herbs, minerals, or amino acids, or they had to get a doctor's prescription for testosterone.

With this new opportunity, however, has come a great deal of confusion and misinformation. The confusion is easy to understand. There are three different classes of T-boosters, and each has several types. To make matters worse, the names of the various T-booster supplements are, in many cases, very similar, and the same supplement can be known by several different names. For example, androstenedione, the T-booster best known because of the publicity surrounding its use by baseball great Mark McGwire, is also known as "andro" or "adione." It is also sometimes marketed under its scientific name, "androst-4-ene-3, 17-dione."

Then there is an entire class of "nor" T-boosters whose names mimic the names of others except they are preceded by the prefix *nor*. Thus, the T-booster 4-adiol and androstenedione have their "nor" counterparts, nor-4-adiol and nor-androstenedione. The latter is also known as nor-androstenedione, 19-nor-androstenedione, and 19-nor-4-androstenedione.

Why the confusing names? Why couldn't the T-booster manufacturers come up with something cute or catchy like Viagra? Well, unlike pharmaceuticals, which are released with huge marketing budgets by giant drug companies, T-boosters don't belong to any one company, so no one, in effect, has the right to name them. Their current names are abbreviated versions of their scientific names. Viagra's scientific name is "sildenafil citrate," which isn't much more memorable than androstenedione.

Misleading advertising has compounded the confusion. Some disreputable supplement companies have purposely taken advantage of the newness of T-boosters to market non-T-booster products as having the same attributes. Don't let this keep you from benefiting from these remarkable supplements.

As previously mentioned, the T-boosters can be divided into three categories: testosterone precursors, nor-testosterone precursors, and miscellaneous. T-boosters, or testosterone prohormones, convert to testosterone in the human body via a single chemical step. Nor-testosterone boosters don't convert to testosterone but instead get transformed into nor-testosterone, which is a potent biochemical cousin of testosterone that is best used for fast fat loss and muscle gain. It is not very effective in enhancing sex drive, and in many cases it may even dampen sexual interest by acting like the female hormone progesterone. On the other hand, the nor-T-boosters have fewer androgenic or masculinizing side effects (acne, hair loss in men or body hair increase in women, and prostate stimulation) than testosterone. Let's take a closer look at each category.

Category 1 T-Boosters: Testosterone Precursors

Androstenedione (Adione)

Androstenedione is biochemically synthesized from DHEA and 17-hydroxy progesterone in the testes, ovaries, and adrenal glands, which sit on top of the kidneys. Androstenedione was the first T-booster to become available over the counter in 1996, but it had been synthesized decades earlier. In 1936, Dr. Charles Kochakian was the first to show that it had both androgenic (masculinizing) and anabolic (muscle-building) effects.

Androstenedione has been widely publicized and used even though it is not a very strong T-booster. When Mark McGwire admitted in August 1998 to using it regularly, the resultant hysteria underscored the public's—and, more troubling, the medical profession's—lack of understanding of T-boosters. Rather than rationally examining androstenedione and its related testosterone precursors, androstenedione was immediately labeled a "dangerous steroid," which was inaccurate on both counts.

When biochemist and bodybuilder Patrick Arnold first introduced androstenedione, initially only one small supplement company would sell the product. Two years later almost all the major supplement companies have jumped on the bandwagon and sell their own versions.

Since its introduction, an estimated 50 million doses have been taken by consumers with no reported adverse side effects. I myself have probably consumed about three hundred of the 100-milligram capsules of androstenedione and two hundred capsules of the 100-milligram doses of 4-adiol (I average about one a day of each) without noticing any adverse effects over the last twelve months.

Now compare that safety record with Viagra. During its first year of use, according to the Food and Drug Administration, 130 recorded deaths were associated with its use. That is not to say that Viagra caused all the deaths. Most, if not all, of the men who died were in poor health and had preexisting life-threatening conditions. The point, however, is that by any reasonable standard androstenedione and its related T-boosters are safe.

Like all T-boosters, androstenedione is a naturally occurring hormone in the human body. It is abundant but relatively inactive until it converts into other hormones. Androstenedione is a T-booster since it is only one chemical reaction away from converting to testosterone in the human body. However, it should also be considered an "E-booster" since it can also be converted first into an estrogen known as estrone. By another single step it can be further converted into the commonly known estrogen estradiol.

An East German study on androstenedione showed that it can increase testosterone levels up to 250 percent, although research shows much less of a testosterone-boosting effect. One study conducted in 1997 by Muscle Media 2000, a major sports nutrition company, measured the baseline testosterone levels of eight healthy, male weight lifters. Four of the men were then given a placebo, and the other four a supplement mixture that included 80 milligrams of androstenedione. Within ninety minutes the men receiving androstenedione had an average increase in testosterone levels of 24 percent, while the placebo group's testosterone levels actually went down slightly. The test subjects were told to continue taking either androstenedione or the placebo twice a day for two weeks. At the end of the study, baseline testosterone levels were measured and were found to be virtually the same in both groups. Judging from this small study, it appears that androstenedione raises testosterone levels in the short term but has little effect on testosterone in the long term.

In a more recent study, presented at the International Congress of Weightlifting and Strength Training in Finland in 1998, seven men, ages twenty-two to thirty-three, were given 100 milligrams of androstenedione. The average increase in total testosterone levels after ninety minutes was 14 to 16 percent higher than their baseline levels.

The effects of androstenedione on women have been studied as well. It is important to note that a normal young woman makes about 45 to 50 micrograms of testosterone a day, whereas a young healthy man makes about 5,000 to 7,000 micrograms. This means a man makes at least one hundred times more testosterone daily. A woman's blood serum contains from 20 to 80 nanograms per deciliter (ng/dl) of testosterone, whereas a man has 250 to 1,000 ng/dl. So a small amount of increase in a woman's testosterone levels has a bigger impact because there is so little to start with.

I usually give my women patients who are fifty years of age and older 1 to 5 milligrams of a testosterone transdermal gel daily, whereas the men get 25 to 100 milligrams daily for medical androgen deficiency. As women's ovaries cease operating due to aging or medical or surgical menopause, the adrenal glands become the major source of androgens by producing androstenedione, which is transformed into testosterone outside the adrenal glands.

A scientifically sound, double-blind study on androstenedione's effects on women was conducted in 1980 by medical researchers John Bancroft and Niels Shakebaek. Fifteen young women who complained of low sex drive due to oral contraceptive use were given a small daily dose of 20 milligrams of androstenedione for two months. There were no reported adverse side effects.

Most women on birth control pills containing estrogen will have a drop of sexual interest because the resulting increased estrogen decreases the availability of free testosterone. For those wishing to "spike"—that is, temporarily elevate—their testosterone levels, androstenedione may be a good choice. It is economical and readily available. However, since it can also spike estrogen levels, women may wish to take another T-booster that cannot convert directly into estrogen.

4-Adiol (4-Androstenediol)

The second T-booster developed and introduced in the marketplace is a somewhat obscure hormone that occurs naturally in animals, including humans, in very small quantities. It is found in the uterus, testicles, adrenal glands, hypothalamus, and pituitary gland. Despite the intense media attention that androstenedione has received, 4-adiol is actually a much more potent testosterone booster.

A 1998 study led by Timothy Ziegenfus, a researcher at Eastern Michigan University, revealed that a single dose of 100 milligrams of 4-adiol can increase testosterone levels by 50 percent or more over baseline levels. The conclusion reached was that 4-adiol is three or more times more potent than androstenedione in elevating T levels in men. Just think what 4-adiol could do to women's T levels! Another study showed that 4-adiol converts to testosterone three times greater than androstenedione converts to testosterone.

Another advantage that 4-adiol has is that it cannot convert directly to estrone and then to estrogen, as androstenedione can; its biochemical structure converts mainly in the direction of testosterone. Those who have issues about excess estrogen levels may want to consider the use of 4-adiol instead of androstenedione. Another consideration, however, is that at present 4-adiol is about twice the price of androstenedione.

•➤ *Caution:* Toxicity and long-term studies have not been done yet on 4-adiol. It is recommended that low doses be taken infrequently unless natural androgen levels have been depleted by age, disease, or a medically diagnosed condition.

5-Adiol (5-Androstenediol)

While technically classified as a testosterone precursor, 5-adiol is highly unlikely to produce significant increases in testosterone levels. The body does convert 5-adiol to testosterone, but in extremely small amounts (less than 1 percent of the total dosage of 5-adiol). Beware of any manufacturer selling 5-adiol and touting it as a testosterone booster. This is not to say that 5-adiol is useless. It can convert back to DHEA (from which it originates), which has other health benefits as mentioned in the previous chapter. In addition, animal research suggests that 5-adiol may have potent effects at enhancing and balancing the immune system. A 1992 study at the Medical College of Virginia showed that 5-adiol was extremely potent at boosting immunity in mice, at least against a certain virus. Whether this effect will be as strong in humans has not been proven.

A Central European study that examined the effects of 5-adiol and other hormones on rats showed a mild anabolic effect, although significantly less than that of 4-adiol and methyl testosterone. This mild anabolic effect may be a reason for its use as a veterinary steroid in foreign countries, but there has been little research done on humans.

Category 2 T-Boosters: Nor-Testosterone Precursors (19-Nor-Testosterone)

By altering the chemical structure of testosterone slightly, a compound is created called nor-testosterone. In medicine and pharmacology, the nor-T compounds are often referred to as the "nandrolone family," or the "nor" version of testosterone.

All three Category 1 T-Boosters can be altered in the same way to become nor-testosterone boosters. For example, the testosterone booster androstenedione has an equivalent nor-testosterone booster called nor-androstenedione, and the equivalents for 4-adiol and 5-adiol are nor-4-adiol and nor-5-adiol.

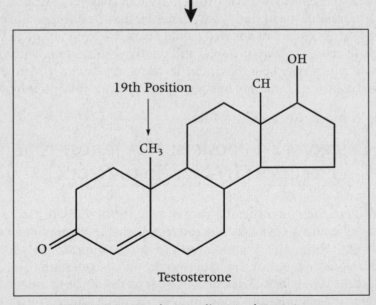

17th Position ⟶ O

CH

CH₃

Androstenedione

19th Position

CH

OH

CH₃

O

Testosterone

FIGURE 2—*Androstenedione and Testosterone*

When deciding which anabolic hormone to prescribe, a doctor often looks at the anabolic-to-androgenic ratio. This ratio roughly measures how much muscle growth a hormone induces (anabolic) compared to how much masculinizing or sexual enhancing side effects (androgenic) it could generate. The anabolic-to-androgenic ratio of testosterone is one to one. In other words, it is as anabolic as it is androgenic. But the anabolic-to-androgenic ratio of nor-testosterone has been measured in several different studies and is estimated to be ten times more anabolic than androgenic. Thus, nor-testosterone compounds are considered ideal for gaining muscle with less or minimal androgenic side effects. This is why bodybuilders love it.

However, nor-testosterone does not improve libido and can actually suppress it. And like testosterone, nor-testosterone will also shut down your natural testosterone production if taken for a long time without periodic breaks.

•➡ *Caution:* The nor-T agents can increase risk to the cardiovascular system and can lower HDL cholesterol levels significantly since their novel structure allows them to minimally convert to estrogen. Persons with existing heart conditions should avoid taking nor-T (Category 2) agents.

Nor-Androstenedione (Nor-Adione)

Also called 19-nor-androstenedione or 19-nor-4-androstenedione, the "nor" version of androstenedione has the same properties except that it converts to nor-testosterone instead of testosterone. It can also convert to estrogen just as androstenedione does, but at a much lower rate.

Unlike androstenedione, it may actually lower estrogen levels in both sexes, although the research on this is not conclusive. This product was introduced to the market as an alternative to androstenedione; it has fewer androgenic (masculinizing and libido side effects) and more anabolic (muscle-building) effects. You won't experience an increase in sex drive after taking nor-adrostenedione, but you may have increased energy as well as accelerated fat loss and muscle gain.

Many supplement companies have marketed nor-androstenedione as the natural over-the-counter alternative to Deca-Durabolin, the extremely popular, medically prescribed anabolic steroid that contains nor-testosterone. While nor-androstenedione is an effective nor-testosterone booster and can be of benefit to those seeking a better body, its effects are not nearly as strong as those of the pharmaceutical anabolic nor testosterone steroids, which are illegal to possess without a doctor's prescription.

Nor-4-Androstenediol (Nor-4-Adiol)

This is the most recent prohormone introduced to the supplement market. Like 4-adiol, the direct testosterone precursor, this supplement is also extremely potent. While it just became available as a supplement in the United States in 1998, it has been sold in foreign countries for many years as the anabolic steroid Bolandiol.

Only 4-adiol can compare with nor-4-adiol in terms of potency of over-the-counter prohormones. Just as 4-adiol will deliver a large increase in testosterone, nor-4-adiol will deliver an equally large increase in nor-testosterone. Although not good as a libido enhancer, nor-4-adiol is perhaps the best T-booster for those serious about gaining muscle and losing fat. In bodybuilder circles, it's known as the "nun" or "monk" T-booster because of its asexual effect. Indeed, nor-4-adiol could decrease capacity in male erection over time and decrease vaginal lubrication. There is some evidence that it might even shrink testicles if taken over a long time without periodic breaks, and this can affect sexual performance and fertility—the price extreme bodybuilders pay for taking substantial amounts of nor-4-adiol to acquire big musculature.

•← *Caution:* Like nor-androstenedione, nor-4-adiol is not recommended for those with a personal or family history of heart disease or depression.

Nor-5-Androstenediol (Nor-5-Adiol)

The chapter on this prohormone has yet to be written. We know that it does convert to nor-testosterone in very small amounts, but it may also have estrogenic effects. Care should be taken when purchasing a nor-4-adiol product that nor-5-adiol isn't purchased accidentally. Several small companies are selling nor-5-adiol as a body-building supplement, but none of them have presented any research that suggests it has any positive effect whatsoever.

•➔ *Caution:* This supplement is not recommended until more research has been done and definitive information about its effects is available.

Category 3 T-Boosters: Phyto- and Pseudo-T-Boosters

At the same time that testosterone prohormones were introduced in 1996, several other products came on the market claiming to boost testosterone levels and increase both muscle mass and libido. Most of these products are not pro-testosterone hormones and include various herbs and plant extracts that are supposed to enhance the body's anabolic hormonal balance.

Tribulus Terrestris

This ancient Indian herb has long been used to enhance sexual drive in both India and China. A Bulgarian pharmaceutical company called Sopharma has been selling it for decades as a testosterone booster for medical purposes, originally for infertility therapy. A formula with tribulus and other herbs was sold in Eastern Europe under the trade name Tribestan. After a strong underground following among bodybuilders brought it to the United States, Sopharma licensed the formula to several American supplement companies for sale here.

The company claims to have done several studies on Tribestan that showed increases of up to 30 percent in testosterone levels of men. Tribestan also reportedly increased men's libido, strength of erections, and sperm production. Effects reported on females include increased estrogen levels, libido, and fertility. But this research has yet to be published in the United States and face scrutiny from the Western medical community.

If this research is in fact legitimate, tribulus may be a good alternative or an adjunct supplement to androstenedione or 4-adiol. While androstenedione or 4-adiol converts directly to testosterone, tribulus is reputed to cause the release of a pituitary gland hormone called luteinizing hormone (LH), which sends a message to the Leydig cells in the testes to produce more testosterone.

Taking androstenedione or 4 adiol for too long may eventually cause the body to shut down production of LH, so tribulus may be helpful if used along with other T-boosters. However, caution should be used regarding tribulus until the Bulgarian studies are replicated by Western scientists and published in a peer-reviewed, scientifically credible medical journal.

My clinical experience with tribulus in elevating LH or testosterone in my middle-aged male patients has been disappointing. Herbal agents such as tribulus appear to be too weak to benefit an aged hypothalamic-pituitary-gonadal system. The better effects would seem to be in young people who have well-functioning hypothalamic-pituitary systems. The other problem is the relatively high cost (in comparison to T-boosters) and the need for doses twice what is recommended.

Chrysin

This naturally occurring substance belongs to a family of compounds called isoflavones (phyto-estrogenic compounds) that are found in soybeans, flax husks, red clover, and other plants. Chrysin is found in a species of passion flower called *Passiflora coerula*.

Its entry into the supplement market was highly anticipated due to a 1996 article in a fitness magazine by health guru Dan Duchaine. He wrote that the information he was about to present "may be some of the most important writing I've ever done. Its applications will profoundly influence a man's body from puberty until death. By manipulating naturally occurring estrogen in the male metabolism, an individual will allow greater height gains during adolescence, raise testosterone production to 30% over normal, and postpone the declining testosterone secretion that occurs from middle age onward."

Although it was clear he was referring to chrysin, he didn't mention it by name, further adding to its mystique. With this type of fanfare, many bodybuilders and antiaging enthusiasts were eager to get their hands on the substance. Duchaine's enthusiasm for chrysin was based on *in vitro* research that showed chrysin was as effective in inhibiting the conversion of testosterone to estrogen as some prescription anti-estrogen drugs called aromatase inhibitors.

If chrysin worked in the human body as well as in a test tube, it would be a good supplement for safely elevating testosterone levels and preventing some undesirable side effects of estrogen. But that's a big if; research in the lab frequently does not translate to the real world. No studies have yet been published on orally ingested chrysin. Until further research is done, this supplement's effectiveness is still in question.

Ipriflavone

Ipriflavone has a chemical structure that resembles the estrogen-like isoflavones found in lentils, beans, chickpeas, soybean products, and whole grains. Most research on this synthetic compound has been on its bone-building properties, but a Hungarian pharmaceutical company, Chinoin, conducted research that showed possible muscle-building effects. According to the company's patent on Ipriflavone, administration of this supplement caused muscle gains of 7 to 20 percent in many different animals. Whether Ipriflavone will have this effect in humans still hasn't been determined.

One U.S. company is selling this supplement as part of a combined formula with tribulus to increase testosterone. In theory, Ipriflavone may act to block potent estrogens like estradiol or possibly slow the conversion of testosterone to estrogen. For the moment, however, the research remains inconclusive. Ipriflavone is sold as a drug for increasing bone mass and for treating osteoporosis in such countries as Japan, Hungary, and Italy.

7-Keto-DHEA

This naturally occurring hormone is closely related to DHEA. It has been researched extensively by Dr. Henry Lardy of the University of Wisconsin, Madison, in cooperation with the Humanetics Corporation. One sports nutrition company is marketing this supplement as an alternative to androstenedione, claiming it will increase muscle mass without any androgenic side effects.

However, there is at present no evidence whatsoever that it will increase muscle mass. In fact, one study showed that it might have the opposite effect. In this study, 7-keto DHEA was given to eighteen healthy men and a placebo to six men, ages eighteen to forty-nine, over an eight-week period. At the end of the study, testosterone levels were actually slightly lower in the men taking 7-keto DHEA. Thus, it appears unlikely to be a good supplement for building muscle.

It does show promise as an immune system enhancer or regulator. Research by Lardy shows that 7-keto DHEA may stimulate the production of interleukin 2, which is an important factor for helping the immune system. This supplement could be a valuable tool to prevent and treat viral conditions like the common cold or flu.

In another study by Lardy, mice given 7-keto DHEA were better able to remember directions through a maze than a control group. Whether it will have the same effect on human memory remains to be seen.

Since 7-keto-DHEA does not convert to testosterone or estrogen, it is unlikely to increase muscle mass or libido. An overall recommendation cannot be given since there are not enough data available. Watch for possible future data on its immune function.

Take It Home

While many products are promoted as sexual enhancers, particularly those sold on the Internet, most of them are essentially herbs with only an indirect, if any, effect on testosterone levels. For a T-booster to work effectively, it must elevate testosterone.

In the last two years, six separate Category 1 and Category 2 T-booster products have been developed, so it might seem that there could be a never-ending stream of new ones. That's not likely. Most of the natural testosterone biochemical pathways have been discovered. What we can look forward to is additional research that will refine the use of currently available T-boosters.

Part II

The Natural Body Makeover

· 4 ·

How to Lose Fat Naturally

The problem with most diets is that you lose both fat and muscle when you lose weight. Muscle is the most active lean tissue and burns calories much faster than fat tissue, so it's the last thing you want to lose in a weight-loss program. The idea is to be lean—that is, muscular—not just thin. Without adequate muscle mass, any dieter is doomed to failure.

This is the beauty of using T-boosters in a weight-loss program: They help ensure that more of the weight loss comes from fat rather than muscle. In this regard, T-boosters are truly an innovation: There is nothing else that can make that promise. But it gets better. Not only do T-boosters allow you to retain current lean body mass, but they can even *increase* your muscle tissue and metabolism while you are losing weight.

In this chapter you'll discover how natural supplements in combination with a dieting and exercise regimen called "cycling" can allow you to shed extra pounds of fat. Before discussing how to use T-booster supplements in a weight-loss program, though, it is important to review why most diets don't work.

Efficient Fat-Burning Machine

Gaining more muscle means an increase in resting metabolic rate— the rate at which the body consumes calories for energy while at rest. Every pound of muscle gained means 30 to 50 more calories a day burned off without exercise. This is equivalent to losing from three to five pounds of total body weight for every pound of muscle added in a year's time.

By now most dieters know that a proper weight-loss—or, rather, fat-loss—program is not about pounds but inches. Muscle weighs more than fat. The goal is "recomposition." You want to turn your body into a healthier version of its old self—a new lean and fast fat-burning (fat-oxidizing) machine. And this has nothing to do with age. Numerous scientific studies have shown that a body makeover can by done at virtually *any* age—even into your eighties—with the proper regimen of hormone balance, supplements, diet, and exercise.

A gain of five to ten pounds of muscle can be a tremendous help in burning calories. As you gain more lean muscle mass, you become a more efficient fat-burning machine for every calorie you consume. You also become more efficient in building energy molecules called ATP. In a paper presented at the 1998 Endocrine Society's annual meeting in New Orleans, Dr. R. Leibel explained that a group of obese men and women were put on low-resistance bike exercise to measure how they burned calories. Surprisingly, despite their excessive fat, they utilized more carbohydrate calories for energy than fat calories. On the same bikes at the same low-resistance settings, the results were the opposite for a group of lean men and women. Most of their energy came from fat. Ironically, the study concluded that the obese person is less efficient than the lean person in utilizing the most dense energy form—fat molecules.

Unfortunately, with most weight-loss programs that simply restrict calories, muscle mass as well as fat tissue is lost. If only you could tell your body to lose fat rather than muscle the next time you skip the chocolate cake. When you're overweight, though, your body does not discriminate as to the type of body mass it loses.

The Right Combination of Exercise

The right food intake can help you maintain current levels of muscle. A diet high in lean sources of protein and low in fat and simple carbohydrates is better than one in which calorie intake is reduced without any thought of food groups. Lean protein sources include egg whites, skinless white meat chicken, fish, protein powder from plants, and milk extracts. (See Appendix 1, Table 2.)

To build more muscle, you need to incorporate weight training into your exercise program two or three times a week. Recent studies have shown that combining intense or anaerobic exercise with low-intensity exercise achieves greater weight loss overall than low-intensity aerobics alone.

Exercise is important because only a small amount of the calories consumed is used to process the food intake. The vast majority of the one million calories that the average person consumes annually—65 percent—is used by your resting metabolic rate. This is the energy the body needs for basic operations and maintenance such as cell formation and repair, breathing, heartbeat, and muscle tone needed for sitting, standing, and so on. The rest of the food calories are used during physical activity. The result is that the more physical activity in which you engage, the more calories you burn. But the *type* of physical activity is as important as the *amount*.

The best combination of exercise for a body makeover combines aerobic with anaerobic in a regimen of sixty to ninety minutes at least three times a week. The anaerobic exercises are ones in which you have to stop and "catch your breath." It doesn't really matter how you get out of breath. What counts are an increased heart rate, an increased demand for oxygen by the cells, and a buildup of lactic acid.

A good exercise regimen is to alternate two to five minutes of high-intensity exercise with ten to fifteen minutes of low-intensity exercise. Do what feels most comfortable at first and then always advance your routine in small increments. If you are considerably overweight, then wait until you have lost some weight before doing any intense "impact" type of exercise such as running, stair climbing, jumping, or hill climbing. This will protect your joints from getting inflamed.

Here are examples of high- and low-intensity types of exercise:

High Intensity (Anaerobic)

Running or sprinting
Stair or hill climbing

High-resistance biking (uphill)
High-resistance pedaling on a stationary bike
Power walking (need to stop or slow down to catch your
  breath)
Lindy hop, swing or tango dancing

Low Intensity (Aerobic)

Easy level-ground walking
Gentle jogging
Easy weight lifting with frequent pauses
Mellow fox trot dancing
Gentle reggae dancing
Pedaling on a stationary bike with no resistance

Why the mix of exercise types? Because the most efficient way to build muscle mass and metabolic efficiency is to work all the different parts of your fat-burning machine. It is easier to increase muscle mass if the body as a whole becomes leaner rather than just one part, such as the biceps. You'll also look better if your musculature develops all over rather than in isolated areas.

If you are very overweight or have done no exercise training in more than six months, you should begin with a total of twenty to thirty minutes of a mixed exercise routine and slowly work up to sixty or ninety minutes over the course of six to eight weeks, or what feels right to you. Start at 50 to 60 percent of your maximum heart rate for the low-intensity part and then do a few minutes of exercise that just puts you out of breath. Push the high-intensity part later. The initial goal is to get in the habit of exercising every other day or at least four or five times weekly.

The T-Booster Edge

How should you incorporate T-boosters into your fat-loss program? In a general way, T-boosters can help modify the negative effects of dieting. Restricting caloric intake makes many people feel a little weaker and sometimes a little grouchy. T-boosters will reenergize and improve your mood so that you will want to increase your exercise and stay on the fat-loss program.

Restricting caloric intake can also lower the capacity to synthesize testosterone. Most overweight people (body mass index greater than 26-27; see Appendix 1) who have an expanded waistline also have an excess of cholesterol and other bad fats called LDL cholesterol. Very obese men with waists that hang over their belts usually have a lot of fat stored inside the belly (visceral adipose tissue). A high percentage of these men have low testosterone levels and also have a higher risk for diabetes, stroke, and heart disease. This is also true for women with excessive intra-abdominal fat, or fat above the hips. T-boosters are a safe, easy, and effective way to start to counteract these adverse effects of dieting. If you are in good health, you can take T-boosters two or three times a week before your most intense workouts.

One Cycle at a Time

Cycling is the most effective way of maximizing the T-booster edge in a fat-loss program. By cycling I mean adjusting your diet-exercise-supplement regimen from time to time. The reason for cycling has to do with the body's innate and ancient need to normalize changes encountered in its environment in order to preserve the species.

Losing weight in Paleolithic times meant the loss of capacity to reproduce, so the human body evolved with an ingenious mechanism. Whenever there was a marked restriction in calories, the body's metabolism would automatically slow down and begin burning muscle mass as fuel. Ingenious, right? Well, yes, if your next meal depended on capturing a four-ton mastodon, but in today's Western culture where food is plentiful, fast, and fatty, it has become an impediment. Obesity is a problem of contemporary man. Paleolithic man had no excess fat to burn. Only in the last two hundred years has there been an excess of calories around to create abundant fat stores—excluding the few thousand fat and decadent Greek and Roman aristocratic types.

If you keep your caloric intake very low, you will initially lose a

lot of weight, but eventually your metabolism will slow down and
you won't lose additional weight. To constantly keep losing fat, you
need to alternate your calorie intake between a low-caloric level and
a determined "maintenance caloric level." This is the minimum
number of calories needed to keep from burning lean mass (muscle
or even bone) for fuel. It is often referred to as basal metabolic rate,
or BMR. Go below it (eat less), and your body reverts back to its Paleolithic origins and begins burning muscle. A medium-frame man
of 200 pounds with an average fat-to-body-weight ratio of 15 percent will have a BMR of approximately 2,400 calories. A medium-
frame woman of 140 pounds with an average fat-to-body-weight
ratio of 25 percent will have a BMR of approximately 1,475 calories.
(See Appendix 1 for more information on determining your BMR.)

Cycling, then, is a means of bypassing the body's natural tendency to keep us nice and fat. Here's how to do it: Three straight
days in a row decrease your caloric intake by 20 percent below your
specific maintenance level (your BMR) while continuing to exercise; after three days bring your calorie intake back up to maintenance for two days. Then repeat the cycle until your desired weight
is achieved. It's that simple. An average-sized man would consume
2,400 calories for two days and then 1,920 calories for three days
before switching back up to 2,400 calories again for two days. An
average-sized woman would switch between 1,475 and 1,180 calories.

Be careful not to go above the maintenance level even though
you may be greatly tempted to do so. If these calorie levels are too
low for you and you feel extremely hungry, try changing your diet.
Avoid the high-glycemic foods that rapidly raise sugar and insulin
blood levels. High-glycemic foods include sugary and starchy items
such as white rice, white bread, cornflakes, corn, and puffed rice
cakes. (See Appendix 1, Table 3, 3rd section, page 198, for a complete list.) These foods will only increase your hunger pangs as your
blood sugar rises quickly and then dips thirty minutes to two hours
later. Instead, increase your intake of vegetables, fruits, and
legumes, which are harder to break down in the digestive tract and
don't result in the extreme peaks and valleys of high-glycemic foods.
High-fiber, low-calorie vegetables and fruits make you feel full from
their water and fiber content with very few calories.

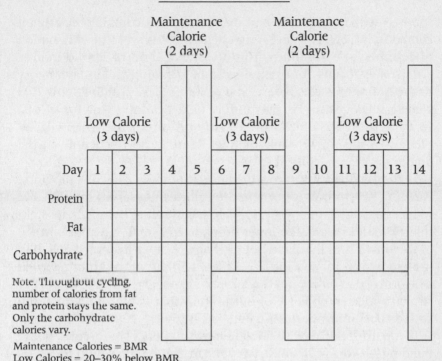

	Maintenance Calorie (2 days)			Maintenance Calorie (2 days)		

	Low Calorie (3 days)			Low Calorie (3 days)			Low Calorie (3 days)		

Day	1	2	3	4	5	6	7	8	9	10	11	12	13	14
Protein														
Fat														
Carbohydrate														

Note. Throughout cycling, number of calories from fat and protein stays the same. Only the carbohydrate calories vary.

Maintenance Calories = BMR
Low Calories = 20–30% below BMR

FIGURE 3 — *Caloric Cycling for Weight Loss*

Paleolithic man ate about twelve servings of a large variety of fruits and vegetables daily and got a lot of fiber, phytonutrients (plant nutrients), and water from them. The average modern man averages two to three servings daily and has an insufficient diet of fiber, water, and phytonutrients. Your cycling diet should include a daily intake of 35 to 40 grams of mixed fibers from fruits, vegetables, and whole grains, both the soluble forms (oats, beans, apples, pears) and the insoluble forms (wheat bran and seeds). This means you need to consume 10 grams of fiber per meal if you eat four times a day or 7 grams if you are on a six-meal-a-day program. The side effect can be excess gas for some people, but a product called Beano can help reduce this effect. In general, fiber supplements are not advisable since they don't have the total health benefits derived from whole foods.

The cruciferous family of vegetables (broccoli, cauliflower, Brussels sprouts) are particularly important because they contain special plant compounds (such as indoles) that help the liver with the elimination of detrimental by-products from the metabolism of sex hormones. Catechol estrogens, for example, can be irritating and inflammatory to the brain, prostate, breast, and other tissues. (Studies show that some catechol estrogens may induce breast cancer.) Aim for at least six to ten servings of colorful low-calorie, antioxidant-rich vegetables and fruits a day while dieting. There is no restriction on the amounts you are allowed to eat.

Lean protein sources are also important for a cycling diet program. Building new proteins burns more calories, preserves muscle, and reduces appetite, and protein is rich in glutamine (which helps fight infection and repairs the inner lining of the small intestine). Much of the time I find that many of my baby boomer patients are low in protein intake. In most instances these patients are attempting to eat a healthful diet by eliminating protein. However, it's not protein per se that's high in cholesterol but protein that is high in animal fat, such as beef, most pork, and dark-meat fowl.

If you are healthy with good kidneys and on a "hard-core" body-building/fat-loss program, try to take in 1 gram of protein for every pound of body weight, ideally spread out over five or six small meals a day, along with a minimum of simple calorie-dense carbohydrates. Thus, a 120-pound woman would want to eat 120 grams of lean protein daily in six meals containing 20 grams of protein each. Examples of small meals with 20 grams of protein are one chicken breast, one-fourth avocado, salsa, one corn on the cob, and one apple; or one small can of tuna packed in water mixed with one tablespoon of low-fat mayonnaise, one piece of whole grain bread, and one cup of red grapes. (See Appendix 1, Table 5, for more food choices.)

• *Caution:* A diet that is very high in protein (more than .5 gram of protein per pound of weight) should not be used if you have any kidney problems or are on medications that affect your kidney function. These medications include the nonsteroidal type of anti-inflammatory medicines such as ibuprofen, naproxen, and ketoprofen. Check with your doctor if you are unsure whether any medication you are taking falls into this category.

Cycling and Supplements

The cycling of low-calorie and maintenance diets will help you lose weight. Adding T-boosters to the formula will accelerate fat loss and reduce cravings, plus give you the motivation to exercise.

In the low-calorie phase of the cycle, men should add 50 to 100 milligrams of Category 1 or Category 2 T-boosters with each meal and/or before each workout, alternating every other day. Women should probably stay with nor-T-boosters at low doses (10 to 25 milligrams) every other day to avoid androgenic (masculinizing) or other side effects.

By using T-boosters during the low-calorie days, your body will burn fat on those days instead of muscle. The T-boosters can also improve mood and energy that might be low on days that you are eating less than you are used to. Some people experience an increased appetite while on Category 1 T-boosters. A switch to Category 2 T-boosters may reduce their appetite.

How and why do T-boosters lead to fat loss and muscle gain? Fat loss occurs partly because fat cells seem to have their own androgen receptors that bind to androgens made from the T-boosters. It is not clear yet exactly how, but the fat cells get the message to break down the fat globules in the cell. The cell's energy factories, the mitochondria, are then signaled to burn fat globules as fuel, a process called oxidation. The fat cell shrinks and may even die.

Androgens also inhibit the fat storage hormone called lipoprotein lipase. Also, Category 1 T-boosters can lower leptin levels. Leptin, a hormonal product secreted by fat cells, regulates food intake by decreasing the appetite of normal people. Men have lower leptin levels than women, probably because they are naturally leaner.

T-boosters also lead to an increased ratio of muscle to fat through other hormonal and metabolic pathways, including the release of growth hormone, a growth hormone–related substance called IGF-1, and other growth factors. Categories 1 and 2 T-boosters also increase muscle mass gain by stimulating protein synthesis.

As with the food intake component of the cycling diet, T-boosters are most effective when used on alternate days. Again, the strategy is to fight the body's natural tendency to normalize and adapt to variations in its energy production. On maintenance calorie days, then, stop using T-boosters to allow your body to reset to its normal hormonal balance.

For best results, continue with this supplement program for six to eight weeks and then stop for six to eight weeks before starting with T-boosters again. This cycle is repeated until you have achieved your desired weight. Again, the idea is to cycle in order to accelerate the fat loss and give your body a rest from the T-boosters.

Thermogenic Formulas

When you have stopped using T-boosters, you may want to try using other supplements to help preserve your muscle gain and keep fat off during dieting. One type of supplement, called a thermogenic formula, usually includes the Chinese herb ma huang, caffeine, and other herbs such as guarana, kola nut, and white willow bark. A quality thermogenic formula consists of a mix of standardized herbal extracts that contains 100 to 200 milligrams of caffeine and 10 to 20 milligrams of ephedra alkaloids (the active ingredients in the herb ma huang and somewhat similar to the decongestant Sudafed). Make sure you buy your thermogenic formula from a reputable firm. Recommended brands include Ripped Fuel, Thermadrene, and Thermogenics Plus.

Taking these supplements two or three times a day during your low-calorie days will help burn fat instead of muscle for fuel and will also help reduce your appetite. It is best to start with a low dose, perhaps one-fourth to one-half the recommended dose on the bottle. If you have never taken a thermogenic formula before, you may experience a strong reaction: Your heart may race and you may feel hot, as if you were having a fever. Don't worry. The stimulation and heat sensation are normal side effects.

Always take your thermogenics with a large glass of water and increase your intake of watery, fiber-rich fruits and vegetables to quench your thirst. If your thirst is not quenched, only then reach for a glass of water. Always try to get your water from water-rich fruits and vegetables first.

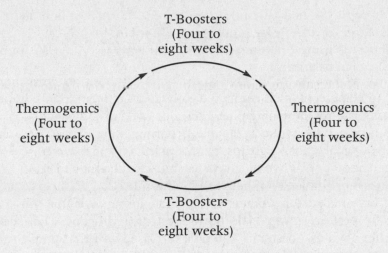

FIGURE 4—*Cycling Supplement for Weight Loss*

•→ **Caution:** Avoid thermogenics if you are sensitive to stimulants or caffeine, or have high blood pressure, heart problems, thyroid problems, or other medical problems that make you sensitive to any type of stimulant—natural or pharmaceutical. Persons in their mid to late sixties or who are ill should avoid thermogenic supplements altogether. Check with your physician before beginning a thermogenic program. Excessive use of ma huang and ephedrine, as well as caffeine and other caffeine sources, can result in heart and blood pressure problems.

In general, thermogenic formulas are safe for healthy and mentally balanced people, and have been proven to be extremely effective. Keep in mind that after several weeks of use you most likely will build up a tolerance. For long-term fat loss, alternate between using T-boosters and thermogenics while switching back and forth between low-calorie and maintenance-calorie days.

Some people may need to use thermogenics and T-boosters together. Since both of these groups of agents are stimulating to the nervous system, you may need to lower the doses of each due to the effect of supplement synergism. The rule of thumb with all new supplements is to start low and go slow—start with low dosages and build gradually to higher dosages.

Women and Fat Loss

Adult women on the average have a body composition consisting of 20 to 30 percent fat as compared to 10 to 20 percent for adult men. That's one reason women have more trouble losing weight—or, to be more precise, reducing fat and increasing muscle mass. (Remember, our goal is not weight loss per se but less fat and more muscle.) To put it another way, women have less muscle than men to begin with, so it is more difficult for them to add new muscle.

The other reason women have trouble losing fat is that they naturally produce fewer male hormones, or androgens. That seems rather obvious, doesn't it? You'd be surprised how that simple truth is lost on much of the medical profession. Physicians frequently prescribe hormone replacement therapy for menopausal women and completely ignore the one hormone that is the most important in maintaining muscle mass—testosterone.

The goal of our natural body makeover for women is to reduce body fat from a range of 20 to 30 percent to a range of 18 to 22 percent, the variation depending on body type. T-boosters can be especially helpful in restoring the natural balance between estrogens and androgens lost with age or, as we will see, from birth control pills.

Estrogen Poisoning Syndrome

The average woman's ovaries stop testosterone production by age forty, well in advance of the cessation of estrogen production. That's right: "Testosterone pause" precedes "estrogen pause" in women by a good ten years. The adrenal gland, another important source of testosterone precursors (T-boosters) in women, also rapidly declines in production by age forty. By ages forty-five to fifty, virtually every woman is androgen/testosterone deficient.

Many menopausal women are so pumped full of estrogen by their doctors that they have estrogen levels higher than in their twenties and thirties—the prime fertile years. I call this phenomenon "Estrogen Poisoning Syndrome." It is characterized by breast swelling, tenderness, and, yes, an automatic weight gain of five to fifteen pounds, mostly in the form of fat.

The problem of excessive fat caused by estrogen overdose is not limited to women over forty. Many younger women also have problems with increased weight and a fatty body composition when they start on birth control pills, which contain estrogen. The type of estrogen in most birth control pills can be four to five times stronger than the type given postmenopausal women.

Excessive estrogen inhibits the body's ability to metabolize carbohydrates, and increases fat storage and hunger. It is another holdover from our Paleolithic ancestors in which the physiological demands of pregnancy, childbirth, nursing, and child rearing required that the excess energy in women be stored in the form of readily available fat.

Besides promoting excess estrogen, oral estrogen pills can also lead to lower "free testosterone" levels—the kind that is available for use. That in turn can lead to diminished sexual desire and activity because oral estrogen pills stimulate the production of sex-hormone-binding globulin, which then decreases the amount of free testosterone available to build new muscle tissue and stimulate the nervous system.

That's not all. Oral estrogen pills can block the positive effects of growth hormone (GH) and its related hormone IGF-1. Together, they have synergistic fat-reducing and muscle-building effects. Also, high levels of estrogen increase a GH-binding protein, so less GH is around.

Alternatives to Estrogen Replacement Therapy

The issue of too much fat aside, overexposure to estrogen increases the risk of breast and other cancers. Unless you have a strong family history of heart disease, osteoporosis, or Alzheimer's disease, estrogen replacement therapy is not necessary at the start of menopause for many women. In fact, without any additional risk of osteoporosis, most women can delay estrogen replacement therapy up to age sixty if there is no family history of Alzheimer's disease or cardiovascular issues.

The most common estrogen replacement pill is called Premarin; the estrogen in this pill comes from the urine of pregnant horses. This estrogen is natural for a horse, and this would be an excellent pill for a postmenopausal horse, but it is not necessarily the best thing for a woman. Automatically prescribing Premarin for any woman with menopausal symptoms is the lazy doctor's way of dealing with a problem that needs an individualized approach.

My recommendation is that you discuss with your doctor the possibility of using natural bi-estrogens or tri-estrogens based on the natural ratios of the estrogens in your body. I prefer that my female patients use transdermal etradiol patches or tri-estrogen or bi-estrogen transdermal creams. I closely monitor the blood levels to make sure that estrogens are in the effective but not excessive range. I also prescribe the so-called weak estrogen estriol (which is produced mainly during pre-puberty) for vaginal atrophy and vaginal dryness.

Often prescribed hand in hand with Premarin is the synthetic progesterone-like pharmaceutical hormone Provera (medroxyprogesterone acetate). Natural progesterone produces a calming effect that can balance the excitatory effect of estrogens, whereas Provera can be irritating and stimulating because of its androgenic-like molecular structure. Many of the synthetic progesterone-like drugs, such as Provera, can promote weight gain and acne, and Provera has been linked to actual increases in heart disease rates.

Provera also antagonizes the effects of testosterone and should not be used together with the T-boosters. To give you an idea of how powerful Provera can be in inhibiting the effect of testosterone, male sex offenders are given injections of Provera to decrease their sexual desire and sexual activity. So use T-boosters in the morning or evening, but do not use them with Provera or other progesterone-like drugs on the nights when you want to feel sexy and are in the mood for some honest-to-goodness lust. Don't underestimate the effect of lust in this body makeover regimen. Sexual activity is a highly effective way of burning calories.

There are many natural herbal and dietary alternatives to the use of estrogen for treating the symptoms of hot flashes, mood swings, and even vaginal dryness during perimenopause or menopause. Among the most effective are phytoestrogens, or plant estrogens, which are found in foods such as soybeans, the lignin in the shell of flax seeds, red clover, and the herbs dong quai and black cohosh.

Unlike human or animal estrogen, phytoestrogens do not increase the risk of breast cancer and do not promote fat storage. In fact, soy products can increase metabolism by enhancing thyroid hormones, which can actively promote fat loss. Both women and men should be careful not to overdose on thyroid as a fat-loss method because too much can lead to osteoporosis.

T-Booster Modification for Women

In general, women can accelerate fat loss by incorporating T-boosters in a diet-cycling program. Women with excessive estrogen because of estrogen replacement therapy or estrogen birth control pills should first consult with their physician for their help in lowering their estrogen levels and simultaneously boosting their testosterone levels.

Do you suspect that your inability to lose weight no matter what you do is caused by hormonal imbalance? Finding out is as easy as taking a blood panel or saliva test. Have your doctor test for the following indicators of hormonal imbalance: total and free testosterone, total estrogens (E1 and E2), sex-hormone-binding globulin, progesterone, DHEA sulfate, free thyroxine index and free T3 and TSH, fasting insulin level, and cardiac risk factor lipids.

The blood level of hormones varies depending on where you are in your menstrual cycle or whether you are in menopause. If your estrogen levels are too high and the free testosterone levels are too low, you will have a very difficult time no matter how hard you diet or exercise.

Take It Home

A regimen that alternates T-boosters, diet, weight training, and high- and low-intensity exercise counteracts the natural tendency of the body to conserve calories and store fat. By increasing your resting metabolic rate, a cycling program incorporating T-boosters will let you overcome those tough plateaus that occur with any weight-loss program.

The T-Booster Fat-Loss Program

Here is a list of the elements to include in your natural body makeover:

I. Calorie-Restricted (CR) Days
  A. Miscellaneous Supplements
    The Antiaging Cocktail supplement below should be used at the lower mid-range limits for younger men and women. Those over 45 can use the mid to higher range.

ANTIAGING COCKTAIL
    Many of these ingredients are included together in multiple-nutrient formulas.
    1. *Antioxidant supplements*
    This group of vitamins, minerals, and phytonutrient antioxidants have been shown in scientific studies to fight one of the leading causes of aging, the production of free radicals, a damaging by-product of metabolism that increases as we age. (IU indicates international unit.)

- Vitamin A (retinol): 5,000 IU
- Natural mixed carotenes with beta-carotene: 5–20 mg
- Natural vitamin E (with gamma tocopherol): 400–1,000 IU
- Vitamin C: 500–1,000 mg, 3 or 4 times daily
- Flavonoid mixture containing:
  - Grape seed extract: 50–300 mg
  - Green tree extract (decaffeinated and standardized): 150 mg, 1 to 3 times daily
  - Mixed bioflavonoid complex with quercetin: 500–1,000 mg, twice daily
- Minerals/metals supporting the antioxidant enzymes:
  - Zinc (chelate): 15–55 mg
  - Copper (chelate): 1–3 mg
  - Manganese (chelate): 5–15 mg
  - Selenium (chelate): 100–500 mcg

    2. *Mitochondrial protectors*
    Every cell in the human body has tiny power plants called the mitochondria that generate most of the body's

energy. With age the mithochondria become damaged for a number of reasons, including exposure to toxic chemicals, leakage of its membranes, and attack by its own or other free radicals. The following agents have been shown to protect the mithochondria from effects of degeneration associated with aging:

- CoQ10: 30–400 mg with food or with vitamin E
- N-acetyl L-carnitine (ALC): 100–2,000 mg before a meal in the morning
- Alpha-lipoic acid: 50–600 mg
- N-acetyl-cysteine: 100–1,200 mg

3. *B vitamins*

The term "B vitamins" describes a group of chemically similar nutrients that are among the most potent anti-agers. Among their reported benefits are the decreased incidence of heart disease, senility, cancer, and depression, and the preservation of memory and the immune system. These nutrients are frequently referred to by their individual names, indicated by parentheses in the following list.

- B_1 (thiamine): 50–100 mg, 1 or 2 times daily
- B_2 (riboflavin): 10–20 mg, 1 or 2 times daily
- B_3 (niacinamide): 20–200 mg, 1 or 2 times daily
- B_5 (pantothenate): 250 mg, 1 or 2 times daily
- B_6 (pyridoxine): 25–50 mg, 1 or 2 times daily
- B_{12} (sublingual methyl cobalamin): 500 mcg, 1 or 2 times daily
- Folic acid (always take with B_{12}): 400–500 mcg, 1 or 2 times daily

4. *Macrominerals*
- Calcium (chelate): 200–600 mg, twice daily
- Magnesium (chelate): 250–800 mg

5. *Trace minerals*
- Chromium (nicotinate): 200–400 mcg
- Molybdenum (trioxide or sodium molybdate): 50–600 mcg

6. *Miscellaneous*
- Betaine HCL: 100–150 mg
- Vitamin D: 400–800 IU

- Vitamin K (phytonadione): 60–300 mcg
- Biotin: 100–300 mcg
- Inositol: 30–100 mg
- Iodine: 50–150 mcg
- Boron: 1–6 mg
- Potassium: 200–500 mg
- Choline: 250–500 mg

7. *Herbs and spices*

Once dismissed as the products of old wives' tales, herbs and spices are now recognized by researchers for their medicinal phytonutrient properties. What's more, food tastes better with them. Use them liberally, but unless you have an unusually spicy diet, you will probably need to take supplements.

- Garlic: 1–2 cloves (4 g), 2 or 3 times daily, or 1–2 capsules (10 mg allin or 4,000 mcg total allin potential), 2 or 3 times daily after a meal
- Season food liberally with cayenne (hot chili peppers), freshly cracked black pepper, turmeric (curry powder), and fresh parsley
- Ginkgo biloba (standardized extract): 40–80 mg, 1 to 3 times daily

8. *Smart oils*

High "lignin" flaxseed oil (refrigerated) or EPA-DHA fish oil: 1–2 tablespoons daily

B. T-Boosters

1. Men under 45 years

50–100 mg of adione once or twice daily, one hour before exercise in the morning. If a second dose is needed, take 50–100 mg after lunch for energy or exercise. Avoid late-night use since it can decrease melatonin levels.

If you are prone to acne or have a hair loss issue, then substitute 50–100 mg of nor-4-adiol once or twice a day. Another option is to use nor-4-adiol in the morning, and 4-adiol after lunch for a pro-sexual and energy effect.

•➤ *Caution:* Do not use the nor T-booster products if you have cardiovascular problems.

2. Men over 45 years

Do not use the nor-T-booster products since they are "cardiovascularly unfriendly" and can decrease libido. Too much adione may aggravate the prostrate or sensitize or enlarge breast tissue in men.

Use 50–100 mg of 4-adiol or adione as described for those under 45. If you want the maximum T-boosting effect, use 4-adiol. For a lesser effect, use adione, which is also less expensive. You could also alternate between the two to see which gives the best effect or take adione in the morning and 4-adiol in the afternoon.

3. Women under 45 years

Women under 45 who are not planning to be pregnant and are not on other sex hormones, including oral contraceptive pills, should use 10–25 mg of nor-adione once or twice daily for the biggest anabolic weight loss effect. For a milder effect, try 10–25 mg of adione once or twice daily.

•➤ *Caution:* Women using sex hormones should not be on a T-booster program.

4. Women over 45 years

For the biggest T-boosting effect, use 10–25 mg of 4-adiol once or twice daily. Take 10–25 mg of adione once or twice daily for a milder T-boosting effect.

C. Thermogenic Formulas

1. Men and women under 45

Take 150–350 mg of ma huang extract (standardized to 6% alkaloids) and 100–200 mg caffeine

2. Men and women over 45

Take 100–200 mg of ma huang extract (standardized to 6% alkaloids) and 50–100 mg caffeine

•➤ *Caution:* Men and women over 45 should be cautious about using thermogenics, especially if they have high blood pressure or thyroid problems.

D. Exercise
- Aerobic: 40–60 minutes, 3 or 4 times weekly
- Anaerobic: 10–20 minutes mixed in with the aerobic exercise
- Total CR exercise: 50–80 minutes, 3 or 4 times weekly
Women need to go to the upper range of exercise time. Age modification: A lower range of exercise time should be used by those over 45 to protect the joints.

E. Sample Meal Plans
The following are examples of appropriate meals to meet daily needs for an average male and female. To modify the program for your specific weight and body type, and for more sample meal plans, consult Appendix 1, Table 6.

Example Female	*Example Male*
Total weight: 140 pounds	Total weight: 200 pounds
Percent of body fat: 25	Percent of body fat: 15
Target daily caloric intake: 1,176 (80% of 1,470 recommended calories)	Target of daily caloric intake: 1,904 (80% of 2,380 recommended calories)
Protein: 60 g	Protein: 120 g
Carbohydrates: 80 g	Carbohydrates: 160 g
Fat: 40 g	Fat: 48 g

Woman's Sample Meals	*Man's Sample Meals*

BREAKFAST

$^2/_3$ cup cottage cheese	$1^1/_3$ cup cottage cheese
1 slice whole grain bread	2 slices whole grain bread
$^1/_2$ cup pineapple	1 cup pineapple
2 teaspoons slivered almonds	3 teaspoons slivered almonds

LUNCH

1 chicken breast half	2 chicken breast halves
$^1/_4$ avocado with salsa	$^1/_3$ avocado with salsa
$^1/_2$ ear of corn	1 ear of corn
$^1/_2$ cup black beans	1 cup black beans

SNACK

2 low-fat string cheeses   3 low-fat string cheeses
1 cup grapes $1^1/_2$ cups grapes

DINNER

3 ounces salmon   6 ounces salmon
$^1/_3$ cup wild rice   1 cup wild rice
lots of green vegetables and/   lots of green vegetables and/
  or salad   or salad
2 cups raspberries   2 cups raspberries

II. Calorie Maintenance Days (CM)
  A. Miscellaneous Supplements
    Same as CR days.
  B. T-Boosters
    1. Men under 45 years:
      Increase T-boosters to the higher range and frequency of use, utilizing the more potent T-booster forms described above in the CR program.
    2. Men over 45 years:
      Increase T-boosters the same way as for men under 45 and utilize the most potent types described in the CR program.
  C. Thermogenic Formulas
    Same as CR days.
  D. Exercise
    • Aerobic: Increase CR exercise duration to 50–70 minutes, 4 or 5 times per week.
    • Anaerobic: Increase CR exercise to 15–20 minutes, mixed in with the aerobics.
    Total CM exercise: 65–90 minutes, 4 or 5 times a week. Women need to go to the upper range of exercise time. Age modification same as for the CR exercise program.
  E. Sample Meal Plans
    The following are examples of appropriate meals for an average male and female. To modify the program for your specific weight and body type, and for more sample meal plans, consult Appendix 1.

Average Female	Average Male
Total weight: 140 pounds	Total weight: 200 pounds
Percent body fat: 25	Percent of body fat: 15
Target daily caloric intake: 1,470	Target daily caloric intake: 2,380
Protein: 75 g	Protein: 150 g
Carbohydrates: 100 g	Carbohydrates: 200 g
Fat: 50 g	Fat: 60 g

Women's Sample Meals	*Man's Sample Meals*

BREAKFAST

²/₃ cup cottage cheese	1¹/₃ cup cottage cheese
1 slice whole grain bread	2 slices whole grain bread
1 cup pineapple	2 cups pineapple
3 teaspoons slivered almonds	5 teaspoons slivered almonds

LUNCH

1 chicken breast half	2 chicken breast halves
¹/₃ avocado with salsa	¹/₂ avocado with salsa
¹/₂ ear of corn	1 ear of corn
1 cup black beans	1¹/₂ cups black beans

SNACK

2 low-fat string cheeses	3 low-fat string cheeses
1 cup grapes	1¹/₂ cups grapes

DINNER

3 ounces salmon	6 ounces salmon
1 cup wild rice	1¹/₂ cups wild rice
lots of green vegetables and/or salad	lots of green vegetables and/or salad
2 cups raspberries	2 cups raspberries

Very Overweight Modification (15 Pounds or More)

Important: Use this program only with the help of a knowledgeable health professional. Even though you need all of the above at a maximum range, the rule here is start slow and low for the exercise part to avoid back, knee, and hip problems and cardiac issues if you are badly out of shape.

Preferred T-boosters: When you are more overweight, you have greater risks of all types of medical problems, especially cardiac and insulin/diabetes and lipid problems. Therefore, use only the T-boosters that are the most "cardiac friendly": 4-adiol and adione supplements. Start at the lower ranges and only after an initial consultation with your physician. The nor-T-boosters are not to be used.

Miscellaneous supplements: The Antiaging Cocktail of supplements at the mid to high AGM (abnormal glucose metabolism) levels is recommended. See page 76.

5

How to Gain Muscle Naturally

One of the most powerful effects of testosterone is its capacity to produce rapid muscle growth. Most people are aware that top bodybuilders and athletes have used anabolic androgenic agents in the past to enhance their physical appearance and performance. The media and the medical establishment have demonized indiscriminately the use of androgens of all types. However, recent medical studies have shown testosterone in its natural form to be an extremely potent muscle-building agent with surprisingly few side effects.

As noted in Chapter 1, the comprehensive study led by Shalender Bhasin, M.D., which appeared in the July 4, 1996, issue of the *New England Journal of Medicine*, revealed that testosterone was essential in gaining lean body mass. In fact, men given the high doses of testosterone, and who did no exercise, gained more muscle than those who took placebos and busted their butts in the gym. But the men who did moderate weight training *and* took testosterone gained almost *twice* the lean body mass as their non-testosterone-supplementing counterparts.

Of course this conclusion was nothing new to the world of bodybuilding. For decades professional bodybuilders had learned firsthand that the quickest way to increase muscle mass and reduce fat tissue was to elevate their testosterone levels in combination with a weight-training program. That's why *synthetic* anabolic agents such as Dianabol, Deca Durabolin, and others were de rigueur in professional bodybuilding circles up until the 1980s. And they were not the exclusive province of bodybuilders. Until they were banned from international competition, anabolic steroids were used by many athletes to become bigger, stronger, and faster than ever before.

The Problem with Steroids

These powerful drugs remain unmatched in their ability to maintain and enhance muscle mass. That's why they continue to be used for patients who suffer from muscle-wasting diseases such as AIDS, multiple sclerosis, Lou Gehrig's disease, and certain anemic disorders. Anabolic steroids work by dramatically increasing protein synthesis and glycogen storage, which are essential for building muscle tissue. These drugs are so powerful that they may allow the athlete to overcome any shortcomings in his training program and still achieve amazing results.

We know, however, that the advantages of synthetic anabolic androgenic steroids come with a heavy price. While some athletes argue it was the abuse of these steroids rather than the drugs themselves that became the problem and that steroids are no more dangerous than many over-the-counter supplements, there is no doubt today that some types pose serious health risks. Among these are an increased risk of heart and prostate disease, liver damage, negative mood alterations, aggressive behavior and sterility. The other problem with these steroids is that they are so powerful they tend to overwhelm the body's own natural manufacture of testosterone. After a while the body senses it no longer needs to produce testosterone, and so production falls permanently. This begins a dangerous spiral of increasing amounts of steroids needed to sustain the previous effect.

New Generation of T-Boosters

The new generation of T-boosters has proven to be safe when used in moderation. There are two differences between T-boosters and synthetic anabolic steroids. Androstenedione and other androgenic hormones occur naturally in the body. In the case of androstenedione, it can even be found in the plant world, in the pollen of Scotch pine trees. Because these occur naturally in the body, the body protects itself from having levels that are too high. These natural T-booster prohormones require the action of protein chemicals called enzymes to be transformed into testosterone or estrogen, or other substances.

As T-boosters circulate in the body, they find specific tissue types with "attraction-type" receptors where the cells transform the inert T-boosters into "active hormones": testosterone, dihydrotestosterone, the estrogens, and other hormones. This process is akin to finding a person you are attracted to that results in the transformational biochemical process called love. Common transformation sites of the prohormones include the liver, skin, breast, prostate, muscle, vagina, bone, uterine-lining cells, and others.

These target tissue sites contain specific enymes for the transformation process. However, there is a limit to what the body can use and transform, which is, in effect, a built-in, fail-safe protection system. The converting enzymes reach a limit of production and can't make more testosterone or estrogen. The excess of the T-booster is eliminated within a few hours, so you can't push your testosterone or estrogen levels to supra-physiological levels with the natural T-boosters the way that you can with synthetic testosterone or estrogen products. Taking T-boosters infrequently further reduces the risk of depressing your natural testosterone production.

The second difference is that injectable anabolic steroids linger in the body for days, weeks, and months, which is why they are easily detected when athletes are tested. The Category 1 natural T-boosters spike testosterone levels for only about three hours. In fact, recently unclassified documents revealed that East German athletes in the 1980s used a nasal spray of androstenedione for a competitive edge during international sports events. Because the testosterone levels were elevated for only a short period of time, the athletes escaped detection and were pronounced "clean" every time.

Some 74 million baby boomers—men and women—experience some degree of androgen deficiency on a daily basis. The result is an increase in fat tissue, depressed mood, increased total cholesterol, and loss of sexual desire. Today, almost everyone who wishes to add a few pounds of muscle to enhance physical and mental well-being can take advantage of the new generation of T-boosters, which are available over the counter in health food stores and via the Internet. Even if you have no desire to bulk up, T-boosters can be used to maintain muscle mass that inevitably diminishes with age.

Training with Weights

Whether your goal is just to remain fit or to get buffed, T-boosters can build muscle tissue when used in conjunction with a weight-lifting or weight-resistance program and an appropriate diet. The term "weight lifting" conjures up all sorts of negative images, such as gyms populated by sweaty muscle-bound monsters, but if you work out at a gym with stationary machines, you already do weight-resistance exercise. Our goal is to maximize that workout by introducing T-boosters into your regimen.

The key to using this new generation of supplements safely and effectively is knowledge. As the saying goes, a little information can be dangerous. In this chapter we'll provide everything you need to know to make intelligent decisions about T-booster supplements for the type of natural body makeover you desire.

Beginner and Intermediate Program

If you are healthy and not abusing any recreational drugs that lower testosterone, such as speed, crack, cocaine, alcohol, or pot, you already have the potential to increase muscle mass without taking any supplements whatsoever. The late, great track and field Olympian Flo-Jo Joyner, with whom I was privileged to work, completely redesigned her physique without the use of any artificial hormone drugs whatsoever, and she revolutionized the training of track and field athletes in the process.

T-boosters can be beneficial even for the beginner by making workouts easier. Any professional athlete will tell you that the hardest part of a new training program is overcoming inertia. T-boosters can help energize and motivate you during the monotony of a workout by intensifying your weight-training program and increasing endurance. The program described in this section is designed to give

that added mental and physical edge with a minimal risk of unde-
sired side effects. It can be used by first-timers or more experienced
intermediate weight trainers and bodybuilders.

Since T-boosters generally give your body a temporary testosterone "spike," they are ideally taken before working out. By taking
T boosters only before working out and no more than three times a
week, you have little risk of side effects, since your testosterone will
have been elevated from its original level for no more than six to nine
hours during a whole week. This spike in testosterone mimics the
body's natural rhythm. Normally, testosterone peaks in the morning
in anticipation of daytime activity and then declines to its lowest
point at night for rest and sleep. Using this approach, you can get
much of the benefits of T-boosters during workouts without the risks
associated with having your testosterone levels elevated all the time.
Because competitive bodybuilders keep their blood levels of testosterone constantly at levels two to three times the upper normal limit
for testosterone (1,000 to 1,100 nanograms per deciliter), they are at
much greater risk for negative side effects. These include the shut-
down of the body's own testesterone production; the conversion of
excess testosterone to estrogen, which can lead to breast growth in
men (gynecomastia) and breast pain and swelling in women (mastal-
gia); irritability and short temper; and possibly the decline of "good"
cholesterol levels. Contrary to popular belief, there is no evidence
that testosterone causes prostate cancer, but it *can* contribute to inflammation, pain, and enlargement of the prostate gland, and promote growth of existing prostate cancer.

If your workout lasts for one hour, it is best to take a T-booster
thirty minutes to one hour before going to the gym Since testosterone levels generally peak thirty to ninety minutes after taking a
T-booster, the maximum brain stimulating effect should occur during the middle of your workout. Testosterone levels will also remain
elevated for about an hour or two after your workout to aid in repair and recovery of stressed muscles and other tissues. If your T-
booster is working correctly, you should experience an increase in
strength, less soreness, and a quicker recovery time.

When using T-boosters only three times a week, you will not experience big gains in muscle mass and fat loss, but you will likely
have better, more intense workouts and beat your previous strength

and fitness records. Continue to use T-boosters three times a week, strictly before weight training, for four to eight weeks.

While it is unlikely that your body will shut down its natural testosterone production if you follow this schedule, it is still prudent to give your body a periodic break. Every third month discontinue taking T-boosters as well as all other hormone supplements, including DHEA, pregnenolone, and melatonin (unless prescribed by your doctor as a medical therapy). This "hormonal vacation" is the same concept as the "cycling" discussed in the last chapter.

Creatine for the Off Months

During the time that you are "off cycle," you can maintain your gains in strength and muscle mass by using creatine monohydrate. Creatine is a natural compound made in the body that supplies energy to muscles. The average person uses 1 to 2 grams of creatine a day, which is about what a sedentary person needs.

The concept of boosting creatine to higher than normal levels to increase muscle building (a process known as creatine loading) was first introduced in 1994 by a team of British exercise physiologists led by Paul Greenhaf, Ph.D. They and subsequent researchers discovered that consuming at least 20 grams of creatine a day could significantly boost muscle mass within one week. The findings spread like wildfire throughout the bodybuilding community, and today creatine monohydrate, the soluble form of creatine, is one of the most popular weight-training supplements. Best of all, because it is a natural substance found in the body like T-boosters, it is legal and safe, even when taken in fairly large quantities.

Creatine monohydrate (or just creatine) supplements are synthesized from the muscle tissues of meats and fish. The highest content is found in the flesh or muscle parts of herring, salmon, cod, cows, and pigs. You would need to eat two pounds of raw steak, herring, salmon, or tuna to obtain the typical dose of 2 grams of a creatine supplement.

In 1998, creatine was wrongfully linked by the news media to the deaths of wrestlers who were severely dehydrated. It was said that since creatine is broken down to "creatinine," a chemically related substance excreted by the kidneys, it contributed to their deaths. While a rise in blood creatinine levels may occur with extremely high doses of creatine, it was never demonstrated that creatine had any causative role whatsoever in the incidents. More likely the reason for the deaths was severe dehydration.

In the medical literature, the only side effect that has been seen with creatine is diarrhea, but only with high dosages (more than 5– 10 grams). Some athletes have complained of muscle cramping. However, a recent University of Memphis study specifically showed that creatine at moderate doses (3–5 grams) did not cause any muscle cramping or diarrhea. The bottom line is that creatine at recommended doses is an extremely safe supplement with a high safety record that can improve strength without affecting hormones.

What is the science behind creatine? It works by providing creatine phosphate to muscle tissue, which allows the body to regenerate the potent energy-producing molecule called ATP (adenosine triphosphate). When muscle tissue contains high levels of creatine, it can regenerate greater amounts of ATP while making less of lactic acid, the nasty stuff that makes you sore and fatigued.

The other positive effect of creatine is that it increases the body's energy capacity to make new proteins, the building blocks of muscles. Muscle building requires lots of energy supply compared to fat, which stores calories very efficiently with very tiny amounts of energy. The more muscle, the less calories will be stored as fat.

Bodybuilders especially love creatine because it increases the volume of their muscle cells by holding in water. This makes muscles look bigger. Beyond the cosmetic appeal, there is evidence that big muscles may be better for cell activity. By increasing the flow of water and nutrients to muscle cells, creatine may also create a nurturing environment for muscles to grow faster.

Creatine monohydrate is extremely popular among professional athletes and fitness buffs because of its immediate effects in increasing strength. This increase in strength, like those produced by T-boosters, translates to a steady increase in muscle mass with consistent workouts.

Creatine is less convenient to take than T-boosters because it must be taken every day to work. Creatine must be stored in your tissues before it can be used as an energy source and before there is a noticeable increase in strength and muscle bulk.

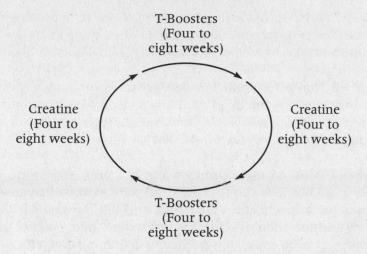

FIGURE 5—*Cycling Supplements for Muscle Gain*

Creatine monohydrate supplements usually come in powder form, to be mixed with water or juice. Most hard-core bodybuilders and athletes typically load up on creatine for five consecutive days by taking 20 grams a day divided in four doses; they then maintain this "loading" dose by taking 5 to 10 grams a day for five days. Recent studies have shown, however, that it may not be necessary to take such high doses. A maintenance dose of 3 grams once or twice daily may be sufficient for a healthy man of average weight (165–185 pounds).

The reason for cycling T-boosters with creatine is that creatine usually increases strength for only eight weeks. After that, most people hit a plateau, so it is best to plan on a four-to-eight-week creatine program and then switch back to T-boosters. Alternating between cycles of creatine and T-boosters allows you to continually increase your strength and performance with minimal side effects.

The Right T-Booster

Which T-booster is right for you? Let's review the three main categories of T-boosters along with their advantages and disadvantages:

Category 1: These have varying degrees of effects in boosting testosterone levels, increasing libido, and building strength and muscle mass: 5-adiol is low, adione is moderate, and 4-adiol is high.

Category 2: Nor-testosterone boosters generally are highly anabolic (strength/muscle building) with low androgenic (masculinizing) effect and little or no libido enhancement. Nor-5-adiol is low, nor-adione is moderate, and nor-4-adiol is high.

Category 3: Most of these products are not pro-testosterone hormones and include various herbs and plant extracts that are supposed to positively affect the body's anabolic hormonal balance. They include tribulus, chrysin, ipriflavone, and 7-keto DHEA. However, more research is needed to determine their efficacy.

If you are a young and healthy male (twenty-five to forty-five years old), it is probably best to start with adione, or androstenedione, since it is the cheapest and most readily available. Adione is a Category 1 testosterone booster and has a medium androgenic capacity. While highly androgenic T-boosters have greater side effects when used frequently, they are the best for producing strength gains after intense exercise cycles.

If you do not get much of an effect from using adione, experiment with 4-adiol, which should produce much higher testosterone levels. This hormone is more androgenic and may be more sexy, producing more of the "male effects" than adione. Thus, it has a higher capacity for sexual drive and protection from heart disease but also has a greater risk of undesirable side effects such as acne and male pattern balding.

If adione and 4-adiol cause acne, sleeplessness, nervousness, or other negative side effects, then they may not be right for your particular metabolism. Switch to nor-adione instead. This hormone, a Category 2 nor-testosterone booster, is less androgenic than the Category 1 testosterone boosters but is less heart friendly and can possibly lower the good HDL type of cholesterol. It also doesn't enhance sexual desire very much. But for men and women with high libidos and strong hearts and blood vessels, the nor-T-boosters may be better. The typical dosage for men is 100 to 200 milligrams taken on an empty stomach or with food one hour before working out.

Modifications to Beginner and Intermediate Program

For Men Forty-five Years or More

The same guidelines apply as for those twenty-five to forty-five years old. However, you should be careful about using the "nor" T-boosting compounds, especially nor-adione and 4-nor-adiol, if you have low HDL cholesterol levels.

• → *Caution:* For men over sixty-five, it is best to use the T-boosters with the help of a knowledgeable physician, since with age there is a greater risk of prostate enlargement, prostrate cancer, breast cancer, sleep apnea (temporary suspension of breathing), and thickened blood caused by increased red blood cells. If you are taking a medication for a physical condition, proceed *only* with the advice of your physician. In general, however, the best T-booster for a healthy older male is 4-adiol.

For Women

Young women in childbearing years need to use caution when incorporating T-boosters into a fitness regimen. No hormones of any kind should be used if you are attempting to get pregnant.

In general, women in their prime fertile years should not use T-boosters more than twice a week, and at low doses of 5 to 25 milligrams. Women tend to prefer Category 2 T-boosters, which have less androgenic or masculinizing effects. Proceed carefully when using Category 1 T-boosters.

Recap of Program for
Beginners and Intermediates

Use this list to keep track of your natural body makeover muscle-building program:

Men Twenty to Forty-five

T-booster cycle (alternate with creatine cycle every 4 to 8 weeks):

> Take 100–200 mg adione or 4-adiol (or nor-adione or nor-4-adiol) before workouts no more than 3 times per week

Creatine cycle (alternate with T-booster cycle every 4 to 8 weeks):

> Loading phase: 1/2 to 1 teaspoon (2.5 to 5 grams) of creatine monohydrate with a sugary drink 2 to 4 times a day for the first 5 days
> Maintenance phase: 2 to 3 grams of creatine monohydrate once or twice daily for the remainder of the 4 to 8 weeks.

Modifications

FOR MEN FORTY-FIVE TO SIXTY-FIVE

Avoid nor-adione and nor-4-adiol if you have low HDL cholesterol, low libido, or cardiac problems.

FOR MEN OVER SIXTY-FIVE

Seek medical advice and medical supervision for modification of the above cycling system of T-boosters and creatine monohydrate.

FOR WOMEN TWENTY-FIVE TO FORTY-FIVE

You should not be pregnant or plan to be pregnant for at least two months when starting this program. Take 10 to 25 milligrams of adione before workouts a maximum of twice a week, or 5 to 15 milligrams of 4-adiol.

FOR WOMEN FORTY-FIVE TO SIXTY-FIVE

Start with 20 to 30 milligrams of adione every other day. If you are not getting results with adione after six weeks, try 4-adiol, 10 to 20 milligrams every other day.

If you have any problem with oily skin, acne, thinning hair, or breast problems, switch to 10 to 25 milligrams of nor-adione or nor-4-adiol. Avoid nor-4-adiol if you have cardiovascular problems.

FOR WOMEN OVER SIXTY-FIVE

Seek medical advice and medical supervision for modification of the above cycling system of T-boosters and creatine monohydrate.

•➤ *Caution:* For anyone on a T-booster program of any kind in this book, *do not* use DHEA, pregnenolone, or other supplemental hormones. The safety and effectiveness of our T-booster program requires you not to add other over-the-counter hormones. Be aware that many sports supplements contain combinations of T-boosters and other hormones such as DHEA and pregnenolone. These sports supplements are not allowed in our T-booster program. The one exception is melatonin in small doses (1 to 3 milligrams). If you are using medically prescribed sex hormones, use our program only under a doctor's supervision.

Advanced Program

For men and women who want a body with a highly sculpted or "cut" look, the moderate approach described above will probably not be fast enough or yield substantial enough results. I'm referring to hard-core bodybuilders or intense fitness buffs who are experienced in weight-resistance training. If you are just beginning to train with weights and are healthy and young, you can make good gains for about two years without any hormone supplementation. However, advanced bodybuilders may reach a plateau where no more gains can be made without supplementation. This is when they often turn to synthetic anabolic steroids to increase muscle mass and enhance muscle definition.

As a medical doctor, I am uncomfortable with the long-term use of synthetic anabolic steroids by young, healthy people. I strongly believe that anyone seeking to use any type of anabolic androgenic steroid should seek appropriate medical supervision because health complications can result. Keep in mind, too, that they are illegal without a doctor's prescription and medical necessity.

Now that many T-boosters are being sold as "legal steroid alternatives," some athletes are using large doses of T-boosters to try to gain muscle quickly, and they are doing it the wrong way. This section is not meant as an endorsement for such use but, rather, as a guideline for the way to get the most results with the least side effects. Most product developers of sports supplement companies are not trained in anabolic steroid biochemistry, nor is the person selling you the supplement in the store. Those seeking to take larger doses of T-boosters may get results similar to those of low doses of synthetic anabolic steroids, but they also increase the risks of the side effects.

You should start an advanced program of T-booster supplementation *only* after knowing the risks involved. In spite of such possible side effects as acne, hair loss, a decline in your testosterone production, sterility, prostate problems, and breast tissue growth, you may still make the choice to attempt synthetic steroid-like gains with T-boosters. Since the elevation in hormone levels from taking T-boosters lasts only three to four hours, you will have to take T-boosters several times a day in order to promote greater muscle growth. Taking multiple daily doses of T-boosters mimics the way the body produces testosterone and its related hormones. Testosterone levels peak in the morning and then go into valleys and spikes throughout the day. By night they drop to their lowest point to facilitate sleep. With age, men lose this testosterone circadian rhythm.

I would argue that taking multiple doses of T-boosters is a better, more natural approach to replenishing testosterone in deficient men than the medically prescribed testosterone patches, such as Androderm and Testoderm, or testosterone injections. The patches constantly elevate testosterone, which is not natural nor desirable, while injections give a much higher than normal level initially, only to crash dramatically later on.

Bodybuilders were the first to use the concept of cycling by rotating various anabolic supplements over defined time periods. They also introduced "stacking," which is the use of a number of agents together to get a synergistic effect. One agent provides what the other doesn't and can act to enhance its effect. As you might suspect, bodybuilders, the human guinea pigs of the underground scientific world, have already begun to experiment with stacking various T-boosters along with other supplements.

The stacking and cycling program below is what I believe will give you the largest gains while minimizing side effects, although you may experience some side effects while on this program or any stacking program. The most potent T-booster in this formula is 4-adiol. This prohormone will give the greatest spike in testosterone and, according to research, will deliver it where you want it most—muscle tissues. Use it no more than three times a week.

Nor-4-adiol is the most potent nor-testosterone (Category 2) booster. Since nor-testosterone has fewer androgenic side effects and is highly anabolic, nor-4-adiol is a good choice for frequent dosing during a "hard-core cycle."

"Hard-Core" Program for Men

Training Days

> Breakfast: Take 100–200 mg nor-4-adiol
> Lunch: Take 100–200 mg nor-4-adiol
> Workout: Take 100–200 mg 4-adiol, 30 to 60 minutes before working out. Take 50–100 mg nor-4-adiol immediately after working out.

Non-Training Days

> Breakfast: 100–200 mg nor-4-adiol
> Lunch: 100–200 mg nor-4-adiol
> Dinner: 50–100 mg nor-4-adiol

•➤ *Note:* Program modifications for men over age 45 and women appear at the end of the chapter.

During the last two weeks or so of your six-to-eight-week cycle, start lowering your dosages gradually. This will allow your body to return slowly to normal testosterone production.

If you think the hard-core program is for you, then before starting have your physician run a blood panel that includes: free and

total testosterone, total estrogens, luteinizing hormone (LH), liver
enzymes, and HDL cholesterol levels. After the cycle is complete,
you should repeat these tests. Do not continue on this cycle for more
than eight weeks without close medical supervision, and take at
least eight weeks off T-boosters or any other anabolic androgenic
hormones before starting another cycle.

An "Off-Cycle" Stack

Some of my patients in hard-core bodybuilding programs have difficulty preserving their strength and muscle gains when they stop
taking T-boosters. This is the result of a combination of physiological and psychological factors. Without the bursts in testosterone,
they do not have as much energy during workouts and are able to
lift less weight and perform fewer repetitions. They become less mo-
tivated and visit the gym less frequently.

The first step in preserving gains is to boost your strength. The best
way without using T-boosters is, as we have said, supplementing with
creatine monohydrate. Start loading on creatine monohydrate a few days
before you stop taking T-boosters. If you load properly for five days, you
can preserve much of your gains in strength and continue to have effective workouts when you come off your hard-core cycle.

Since you were supplementing with T-boosters daily for several weeks,
your body may have responded by lowering your natural testosterone
production; it may even take several weeks for your testosterone levels
to return to normal. One of testosterone's many benefits is that it helps
block the effects of cortisol, a hormone made by the adrenal glands that
induces muscle and other tissue breakdown. If your testosterone levels
are low when coming off a cycle, cortisol can be a major player in the
muscle breakdown process. To counteract this effect, use phosphatidylserine
(PS), a supplement available over the counter. Two studies with a group
of male test subjects by researcher Palmiero Monteleone and his colleagues
at the University of Naples in 1990 and 1991 demonstrated that supplementing with PS before working out can lead to a decrease in the rise of
cortisol of up to 25 percent. Similar findings were achieved in a double-
blind study by Thomas Fahey, Ph.D., of California State University. There
are prescription drugs that can block cortisol almost completely, but they
have proven to be dangerous. Besides, a little bit of cortisol is necessary

for tissue growth. The only way to promote new muscle gain is to stimulate tissue breakdown—but not too much.

Try loading and maintaining PS in the same way as creatine monohydrate. Take 200–300 milligrams of PS divided between two or three times daily with a small amount of fatty food for better absorption. Always take 200–400 milligrams before working out. After one week of loading, you can maintain your PS levels with 200 milligrams twice daily.

When you work out intensely, not only can your cortisol levels rise but your testosterone levels can fall as well. (Weight training can intially increase testosterone, but overtraining will reduce it.) Since your testosterone levels may be lower than normal anyway after a T-booster cycle, you will want to prevent further decline. The quasi-amino acid supplement acetyl L-carnitine (ALC) can help. One recent study indicated that supplementing with ALC before exercise might substantially reduce the drop in testosterone that would normally occur with overtraining.

A study led by endocrinologist Allessandro Genazzani at the University of Modena, Italy, concluded that ALC was successful in bringing sex hormone levels back to normal in deficient women. If you are suffering from lower than normal testostcrone levels due to aging, overtraining, or from overuse of testosterone-raising supplements, ALC may be helpful in restoring your hormone levels.

ALC has other benefits as well. It has been shown to improve mood, concentration, and nerve function, all of which can lead to better workouts. Why? Nerves provide the "electrical juice" for muscle action. The more nerves you can enlist in a muscle contraction, the greater the strength gains. ALC may also help your body use fat rather than carbohydrates or protein as fuel during workouts. Take 1 to 3 grams of ALC a day in divided doses, and always take at least 1 gram before a workout.

Other Hard-Core Supplements

While creatine, phosphatidylserine, and acetyl L-carnitine are the most important supplements to take when you stop your T-booster cycle, there are others to consider. One of these is *Tribulus terrestris*, a natural herbal product that is reported to keep the male body's natural testosterone production high by stimulating the pituitary gland and/or hypothalamus to signal the testes to make testosterone.

Tribulus has not yet been scientifically proven to work, but it is safe and relatively inexpensive. Many medical professionals believe that it requires a well-functioning brain hypothalamus-pituitary-gonadal system for it to work. Men over the age of forty-five may not feel much of an effect. One way to use it is to add 750 milligrams per day to your T-booster stack midway in your cycle. After you have stopped the cycle, increase the dosage to 1,200–1,500 milligrams per day and continue to use it for two weeks.

Other supplements that might be helpful are beta-hydroxy beta-methylbutyrate (HMB) and Ipriflavone, both of which are being marketed by bodybuilding supplement companies. Preliminary research has shown these supplements have potential for building muscle. HMB is an amino acid–like compound that purportedly prevents muscle breakdown during workouts. Several studies have shown doses of 3 grams a day of HMB to be effective, but many bodybuilders say doses of over 5 grams a day are necessary to see results.

Hard-Core "Off-Cycle" Recap

The off-cycle stack for men twenty-five to forty-five years old should include:

Creatine monohydrate: to maintain increases in strength

> 20 grams daily in 4 divided doses for 5 days (loading phase)
> 5 grams daily once or twice daily (maintenance phase)

Phosphatidylserine: to prevent a rise in cortisol, thus preventing muscle breakdown

> 800 mg a day in 3 divided doses for 7 days (loading phase)
> 100–200 mg twice daily (maintenance phase)

Acetyl-L-carnitine: to prevent testosterone decline during workouts

> 1–3 grams a day in two or three divided doses (no loading phase needed)

Optional supplements:

HMB: may prevent muscle breakdown during resistance exercise
3–6 grams a day in divided doses
Tribulus terrestris: may increase natural testosterone production
750 to 1,500 mg daily in three divided doses
Ipriflavone: may increase muscle and bone mass
1–2 grams daily in divided doses

Modifications of Hard-Core Program

For Men over Forty-five

Men over forty-five years may prefer a mix of adione and 4-adiol since nor-adiol may have a negative effect on HDL cholesterol levels. In addition, testosterone levels may have already dropped significantly by age forty-five, especially if you are on certain medications such as some classes of antifungals, antihypertensives, and antibiotics. A better choice for intermittent spiking of testosterone levels for energy, exercise, and sexual boosting if you are already testosterone deficient is 4-adiol or adione.

•➤ *Caution:* The risk of prostate cancer increases as men age. After age forty, every man should have regular digital prostate exams and follow up with a transrectal ultrasound exam of the prostate for any masses or enlargement. A simple blood test called free prostate specific androgen, or free PSA (or "PSA with percent free PSA"), can often be an early detector of prostate cancer. If any doubt exists, have your regular physician refer you to a urologist for a biopsy. Before taking large or frequent doses of 4-adiol or adione, have your testosterone (free and total) and total estrogens (estradiol plus estrone) checked, plus a lipid panel that assesses all the lipids (cholesterol, HDL cholesterol, LDL, and triglycerides) and a blood count (CBC).

I also suggest eating regular servings of soy products and high-fiber vegetable foods on a regular basis. Soy has been shown to have protective effects against prostate cancer and cardiovascular disease. The cruciferous vegetables (including broccoli, cauliflower, Brussels sprouts, and cabbage) are help ful in decreasing cancer risks and excreting some of the "unfriendly" metabolites of testosterone and estrogen.

For Women

Women wishing to embark on a hard-core bodybuilding program utilizing T-boosters should proceed with caution. Never use more than 50 milligrams of any Category 1 or 2 T-booster. The best choice for women may be adione due to its androgenic (masculinizing) activity. Facial hair growth, a deepening of the voice, loss of scalp hair, and acne are signals of excess androgens.

Infertility could be a risk for younger women since T-boosters could act like estrogens and, in effect, prevent ovulation, much in the same way as birth control pills do. For young women in good health and in childbearing years, 4-adiol may be too strong. Younger women may wish to try low dosages of the less androgenic T-boosters such as nor-adione or adione. DHEA might also be an option for women trying to gain muscle since it is one of the weaker androgens available over the counter.

Menopausal women, who need an occasional spike of testosterone, are better suited for the more potent Category 1 T-boosters.

Take It Home

The programs outlined in this chapter are designed for long-term gains in muscle and strength. Most weight-training programs will help you gain at least some muscle and strength, but you will reach a plateau quickly and be unable to make any further gains. The only way to continue to make gains and preserve them is constantly to cycle different supplements and exercise programs. No change equals no gain.

In addition to alternating between T-boosters and creatine, you should also be switching exercises whenever you reach a plateau. See Appendix 3, page 236, for recommendations.

·← Part III ←·

Better Sex

∼ 6 ∼

The Biochemistry of Sex

A recently married thirtyish couple, Joan and Jack, came to my office for a consultation about their sexual problems. The causes of their problems and their subsequent therapy are illustrative of how the chemistry of love and lust differs between the sexes.

Sex had been great leading up to their marriage two months earlier. Now it seemed Joan was no longer interested in lovemaking, at least with Jack, and viewed their sessions as more a chore than a joy. Jack, on the other hand, was very interested in sex but felt like a failure in bed because it was obvious to him that he could not satisfy his new wife in the bedroom no matter how hard he tried. She wanted all warmth and affection. He wanted all wild sex.

Careful medical and sexual history analysis revealed interesting results. Joan's free testosterone levels were subnormal, while her total blood-serum estrogen levels were very high. Jack's test results showed the opposite—low estrogen and a very high free testosterone level. Not surprisingly, the couple greeted the news with a great deal of confusion. Jack immediately insisted they were both perfectly normal. He did not have any estrogen, and he certainly did not want his wife to have any testosterone. After he was through, Joan quietly asked if her beginning the use of birth control pills had anything to do with the problem.

Jack calmed down after I explained that testosterone and estrogen are not gender-specific; both men and women need both sex hormones to function normally. With age, both sex hormones decline, but Jack and Joan, who were both healthy, were still too young to worry about this factor. Joan's question about oral contraceptives turned out to be the answer, or at least part of it.

Shortly before their wedding date, Joan started on a high-potency estrogen type of birth control pill. "We don't want to start a family yet, so I wanted to make sure that I was not going to get pregnant," she said. Being in her prime fertile years, Joan's estrogen was already at peak level. The birth control pills put her estrogen levels through the roof and created an imbalance in her estrogen-testosterone ratio. The testosterone she needed for a healthy feminine sex drive was drowning in a sea of estrogen. The solution was simple: I immediately switched her to a low-potency estrogen contraceptive. She also began taking 10 to 30 milligrams of the T-booster androstenedione one or two times on the day before sex (but no more than once a week) until her sexual interest returned to normal.

Jack's part of the equation was more complex. Jack's testosterone levels were elevated for several reasons. A man's testosterone levels peak in their twenties. Jack was a late bloomer, so to speak. Genetically, he just tended to be at the high end of the range for men. However, he was further elevating his testosterone levels through his diet and lifestyle. His favorite foods were steak, hamburgers, and cheese, all rich in saturated animal fats that promote testosterone production. He got his exercise almost entirely by weight lifting, which, at his intermediate level, also promoted testosterone.

Overloaded with testosterone, Jack had no time for love. All he could think of was sex—a recipe for marital disaster. To readjust Jack's testosterone-to-estrogen ratio, I suggested a diet that reduced his consumption of beef, butter, and whole milk products and included more fruits, vegetables, and soybean products, such as soy "veggie" burgers and soy sausages. The fruits and vegetables helped give a feeling of fullness (he could eat as much as he wanted) and, coupled with the soybean products, balanced some of his excess testosterone. Jack cut back on his weight training and started yoga and prolonged, intense cardiovascular exercises. Before sex, Jack was to take 50 milligrams of nor-adione, a Category 1 T-booster, and then sixty minutes later, 50 milligrams of nor-androstenedione. He was instructed to take the T-boosters only once a week.

Two months later Jack and Joan came back. They were beaming. "Doc, who would have thought the answer to love was to be found in a pill and a veggie burger," he said with a laugh.

In this chapter we will learn *how* T-boosters affect sexual drive in both men and women. Understanding the process will help you enhance the sexual pleasure of both you and your partner. It is also a useful prelude to creating a T-booster regimen customized to your individual profile, which will be explained in the next chapter.

Sex Hormone Primer

A healthy young male in his mid-twenties produces about 5 to 7 milligrams of testosterone from his testes daily. His female counterpart produces about .25 gram of testosterone from the ovaries. A young male, then, secretes twenty to twenty-eight times more testosterone than a young woman.

In both sexes the adrenal glands on top of the kidneys secrete DHEA and androstenedione, which are then converted to active testosterone or estrogen and their metabolites in different target tissue sites such as the liver, skin, breast, bone, prostate, uterus, and vagina.

Blood levels do not accurately reflect the amount of androgen-male hormone activity because of this peripheral conversion of inactive DHEA and androstenedione to the physiologically active testosterone or estrogen. A better measure of testosterone, and its active product called dihydrotestosterone (DHT), is to measure the total male hormone activity. This is achieved by measuring the blood levels of 3 alpha or beta androstanediol glucuronide, which determines the total body level of androgen breakdown products. A woman's serum blood levels of total testosterone can vary between 15 and 80 ng/dl, and the amounts decline with age. In a man the range of total testosterone is also affected by age and health, ranging between 250 and 1,100 ng/dl.

Unfortunately, the doses of T-boosters currently on the market are formulated for a man's requirements. Some T-boosters, such as androstenedione, are sold as 50- and 100-milligram capsules, which cannot be divided easily like a tablet. Studies show that when young women take a 100-milligram capsule of androstenedione, their testosterone can increase a whopping 400 to 700 percent. The male effect was, on the average, only a 15 percent increase in testosterone from the original baseline level.

Women can take some solace in the news that soon to be released are T booster formulations in gel form and in sprays. Once they are proven effective, women can more easily get their appropriate doses. In the meantime, women should use the low end of all dosage recommendations in this book.

Lust for Love

Somewhere in our species' evolutionary development, perhaps between the time walking became upright and the first tool was made, we lost the ability to know when is the best time to copulate to produce offspring. Human sexuality is unique in the animal world in that sex is primarily practiced for recreation, performed on a fairly continual basis and, for the most part, with little regard to procreation. From a biological viewpoint, then, human sex is a colossal waste of time. But then, of course, other species don't fall in love as humans do.

The human sex drive is inextricably connected to our unique ability to love. It is no accident that we call copulation "lovemaking." While other species' sex drives are confined to that period when the female is the most fertile, humans enjoy sex all the time. You might say that because we're in lust continuously, we love. If human sexual pleasure, then, is one part lust and another part love, at its biochemical core are the sex hormones. Testosterone and estrogen— or, rather, their ratio to one another—influence all aspects of human sexuality. A number of factors can upset this balance, ranging from normal aging to environmental toxins and birth control pills.

When taken properly, T-boosters are a safe and easy way to correct this imbalance. Knowing how T-boosters affect the sex hormones is key to mastering their power.

The Sexual Octagon

Based on years of clinically correlating sexual behavior and its relationship to biochemical hormonal tests and events, I have identified eight aspects of human sexuality that are directly affected by sex

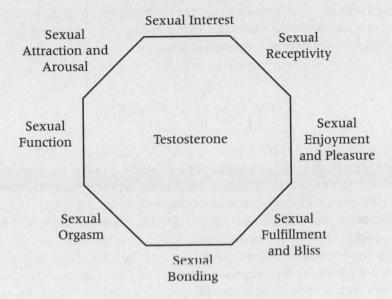

FIGURE 6—*The Sexual Octagon*

hormone ratios. I call this model the Sexual Octagon because all the various facets are interrelated. An imbalance between the sex hormones can affect one or more "sides" simultaneously. The eight aspects are as follows:

1. Sexual interest
2. Sexual attraction and arousal—the lust component
3. Sexual receptivity
4. Sexual function
5. Sexual enjoyment and pleasure
6. Sexual orgasm
7. Sexual fulfillment and bliss—the love component
8. Sexual bonding—love and marriage

As we learned in the case of Joan and Jack, if human sexuality in its eight-sided splendor were not complicated enough, love and lust are often affected by our sexual partner's biochemistry. And just to make things really interesting, women's and men's sexual biochemistry often seem at odds with each other. There is one simple conclusion, however, that science has reached about human sexuality: Without the sexual energy fuel called testosterone, love and lust are impossible to maintain. Let us see how testosterone affects the eight sides of human sexual pleasure.

Side 1: Sexual Interest

The word "libido" is often used to mean sexual interest, but I prefer the latter. "Libido" has all kinds of psychological underpinnings that make it too messy a term from a biochemical viewpoint. The term "libido" was, of course, coined by Sigmund Freud, the father of psychotherapy, who conceived of it as a fixed and finite amount of mind or psychic energy. Today, most scientific sexologists would refer to libido as sexual motivation, governed by a person's "sexual molecular" makeup and influenced by such social factors as religion, ethics, age, health status, and others.

In my clinical practice I am keenly aware of how sexual biochemistry changes in different stages of life. I have witnessed my patients' sexual interest alter as they enter puberty, fall in love, fall out of love, bond and marry, become pregnant, nurse babies, and move on into menopause and andropause. The more mundane events of daily life, such as stress, travel, and illness, can also affect sexual biochemistry.

Sexual interest can be socially influenced and gender specific. A Kinsey Institute study concluded that while sexual activity declined in both sexes with age because of decreasing sex hormones, women's decreased sexual activity was explained at least in part by the lack of available men. Young women on estrogen-containing oral contraceptive pills and menopausal women who take oral estrogens for estrogen replacement therapy both have a dampened sexual interest. Estrogens decrease the level of the active form of testosterone called "free testosterone." The scientific consensus is that the primary force for sexual interest and desire in both sexes is free-testosterone levels. However, a decline in sexual interest does not necessarily have to be preceded by a decrease in free-testosterone levels. Indeed, sexual boredom can be the result of free-testosterone levels that are, well, too boring or too constant. When they remain in a certain narrow, fixed range over an extended period of time, sexual interest becomes less intense.

On the other hand, a quick spike of testosterone such as the kind delivered by a Category 1 T-booster changes the biochemistry of mood. The change occurs mainly through the testosterone-assisted dopamine neurotransmitter system in the brain. When stimulated, this system causes a surge of energy that activates brain memory storage centers. These in turn release and create signals to flood the mind with sexual ideas and fantasies. Where and how the interest is manifested are different for men and women.

Men's sexual interest centers in the brain are thought to lie somewhere in the visual-spatial part of the brain, since men respond so vigorously to visual stimulation—erotic photographs, porno films, and, of course, the female body itself. It is the same reason that men generally do better on visual-spatial tests than women.

Women also feel a surge of brain dopamine-generated energy from a spike in their free-testosterone levels. However, their brain sexual energy is directed differently—more toward areas in the right side of the brain that control abstract thought rather than the concrete literalness of men. This is the same reason that women tend to do better on verbal tests than men. Men create sexual fantasies of the here and now—the proverbial roll in the hay with the farmer's daughter. Women create fantasies of the romantic kind—the gallant Prince Charming who seduces and protects.

Side 2: Sexual Attraction and Arousal

What attracts the two sexes to each other? Here again it depends on gender. Generally speaking, men find women sexually desirable who have a slim waist-to-hips ratio. The exact ratio is somewhat culturally and historically influenced, but the overall ratio appears to be universal and may have an evolutionary basis. Women are most sexually desirable (that is, most fertile) from an evolutionary viewpoint when they are in their younger years. As women grow older and less fertile, their waists tend to become wider.

Of course, middle-aged spread is not limited to women, but stud ies indicate that a man's waistline is not as important a factor in his sexual appeal. Male attractiveness is more difficult to quantify since more abstract attributes such as status and power figure into the formula. Historically, women have found men attractive who can provide for them, and their offspring, although this has changed to some still-to-be-determined degree for Western women with their new economic independence in the latter twentieth century.

Recent research indicates the sense of smell may also come into play in determining sexual desirability. In many animal species, the smell of urine has tremendous influence on sexual signaling and attraction. On some primitive level, do males and females signal each other via odors exuded from their bodily fluid known as pheromones? A recent study showed that women were most attracted to men's sweat-drenched clothes that had the greatest difference in odor from their own odor. From my own clinical experience, this makes a lot of sense. One of the ways I determine if a male is testosterone deficient is to ask him about his body odor. If it is becoming less "pungent" after a good workout or at the end of the day, it usually indicates declining testosterone levels.

The connection between sexual attractiveness and sexual arousal also differs between men and women. For men, they are virtually the same thing—or at the very least there is a very direct, linear association. Men are more dominated by testosterone (free testosterone, that is) and less by cultural expectation and context than women. Men also have larger so-called primitive brain areas that dictate instinctual drives and emotions.

The average woman does not get as quickly aroused when she finds a man physically attractive. However, the more sexually experienced a woman, the less this maxim tends to be true. Previous intense and positive orgasmic pleasure with a man can facilitate arousal. Generally speaking, most women need more from men to be aroused—issues that go deeper than the skin and body shape, including character, confidence, or social-economic status.

There is a third dimension to sexual attraction and arousal—the *capacity* for arousal. Arousal signals in the brain can trigger sexual thoughts, but a physical response may be absent. A man's physiological arousal response—an erection—is relatively easy to quantify. In fact, men, you can even measure your arousal capacity at home with the "postage stamp" test. Paste a ring of postage stamps around your flaccid penis before you go to sleep. If the ring is broken the next morning, it means that you had a normal nocturnal erection and that your penile blood flow system is healthy and intact.

A woman's arousal mechanism is more complicated. Most sex researchers rely on the subjective reporting of vaginal lubrication to measure capacity. However, some women may be aroused but don't lubricate because cells lining the vagina are hormonally depleted or because of poor blood flow to the clitoris.

In men there are sexual arousal nerves in and around the penis, and in women they are in the clitoris, the nipples, and the female "G spot." They are not controlled by the brain but are channeled directly from the spinal cord and back to the sex organs. The nipples will get hard, the penis can become erect, or the vagina may lubricate with simple physical stimulation or sexual thoughts.

Since men's sexual attraction and arousal responses are more directly linked to levels of free testosterone, T-boosters tend to have a more pronounced effect. On the other hand, since women have so much less testosterone than men, an equivalent amount of T-boosters can dramatically spike their free-testosterone levels.

Side 3: Sexual Receptivity

Sexual receptivity means being open to engaging in sexual activity. This requires a certain attitude, a lack of fear or anxiety, and a feeling of security that no immediate physical harm or, over the longer term, damage from infections will occur from sex. As with most aspects of the human sexual equation, how sexual receptivity is interpreted is different for men and women.

For women, sexual receptivity is a subtle "warm and fuzzy" feeling, biochemically driven by estrogen, the primary female sex hormone. Much of female sexual receptive response comes from so-called higher brain activity centered in the neocortex, which also controls the decision-making processes. From a sex hormone point of view, studies have shown that healthy young women are the most sexually receptive when their estrogen levels peak during the menstrual cycle. I call this the yin or estrogen mode, which will be discussed in more detail in the next chapter. In this mode, women are primarily driven by biology, the need to mate. Penetration is more important than orgasm. Shortly after their cycle peaks, women enter a yang or testosterone mode and become more pleasure driven.

Men have a broader band for their sexual receptivity mode since their free-testosterone levels don't cycle monthly or drop off steeply with middle age. Male sexual receptivity relates a lot to the next facet of the Sexual Octagon—sexual function and performance.

In my clinical practice I see a common theme in men in their twenties and older—performance anxiety and fear of infection. Men rarely complain of the physical pain of sex; their greater fear is of the inability to perform well. A mentally and physically healthy male is in a high sexual receptive mode most of the time. He has sexual confidence, which is largely based on his ability to obtain an erection. Performance confidence is what determines male sexual receptiveness.

Viagra has skyrocketed the levels of male sexual confidence and sexual readiness. Before Viagra, I had male patients who faced an asexual lifestyle and sexual isolation because they no longer wanted the humiliation that accompanied their impotency. Newer and even better penile erectile products are just around the corner. However, as close as male sexuality is tied to function, it remains unsatisfying if there is no drive or desire. This is why T-boosters, which fuel the entire sexual energy system, are so vital.

Side 4: Sexual Function

This is the most obvious aspect of human sexuality in which men and women differ. For men, sexual function or capacity means the ability to obtain and maintain penile erection for intercourse and enjoyment. The physiology of erections is all about getting blood into the penis and keeping it there.

Viagra works by knocking out an enzyme that disables nitric oxide. (A UCLA colleague, Louis Ignarro, M.D., received the Nobel Prize in 1998 for his groundbreaking research in this area.) Nitric oxide helps keep blood vessels open and dilated in the penis. This is one side of male sexuality where testosterone does *not* play a role. The male erection can be achieved with absolutely no testosterone. It is well documented that castrated men with very little testosterone in their bodies can have erections.

In women, capacity for function means having an intact vagina and labia that lubricate well and a clitoris that can engorge with blood and become sensitive. Viagra is being studied in older women for its effects on lubrication and overall sexual function. If the vaginal walls are atrophic or paper thin, it will be very painful to have sexual penetration. Vaginal estrogen creams, a 5 percent DHEA cream, or compounded testosterone creams, which are available by prescription, usually can resolve this problem.

Side 5: Sexual Enjoyment and Pleasure

Freud postulated that all our mental processes, especially those in the primitive and primal part of the personality known as the "id," are driven toward pleasure and avoiding pain. He felt that most behavior could be explained by this pleasure-pain principle. This is certainly true in part for sexual pleasure.

Not all sex leads to orgasm, nor is all sex always enjoyable for both partners. Sexual enjoyment must be seen within the context of healthy living and "controlled stress." This will be discussed in detail in Chapter 8, but put simply now, you are not going to enjoy sex if you don't have the energy to do it well. I am referring not to achieving exotic positions but to having a strong physical body and a relaxed, balanced mind. T-boosters can help achieve this goal of better, more pleasurable sex through a better body and mind.

One of the ways that T-boosters increase sexual pleasure is by increasing testosterone levels, not only before but also during sex. Studies on rats (frankly, it's hard to get reliable humans for these studies!) revealed decreased penile sensitivity when deprived of testosterone. Also, the penis shrank in volume when deprived of testosterone. My own patients, both male and female, report an increase of sexual sensitivity and of sexual pleasure thirty to ninety minutes after taking a T-booster, when testosterone levels peak.

Pleasure is hard to define scientifically. It is often equated in the medical literature with not having a sexual dysfunction. My clinical experience leads me to believe that sexual pleasure is like a rainbow—a wide spectrum of colors, each generated by different neurotransmitters and hormones, but activated by the sunlight energy provided by testosterone.

Side 6: Sexual Orgasm

Physiologically, an orgasm can be reduced to a reflex of the spinal cord, and in this sense testosterone does not play a direct role. But we know that sexual orgasm is much more than that. It is the physical *and* emotional culmination of the sexual act. T-boosters play a role by increasing the sexual drive and interest that are the preludes to lovemaking. They also enhance the experience itself.

Orgasm in both sexes involves more systems of the body than any other aspect of the sexual experience. In both sexes, two different nerve systems are called upon: the parasympathetic system (relaxing) and the sympathetic system (excitatory). The parasympathetic system is responsible for erection in males and lubrication in females. The sympathetic system responds differently and comes into play during the latter part of orgasm when the excitement builds, muscles contract, and orgasmic panting, groaning, and spasming occur.

The easiest way to understand the physiology of orgasm is to visualize a series of sensory experiences triggered by spinal cord reflexes. A spinal cord reflex does not involve your brain or any thought. These reflexes are triggered when a certain amount of sensory stimuli reach a threshold level in your spine. Think of water that keeps building up behind a dam. Eventually, the water will spill over. The rush of water over the dam wall is like the "rush" of an orgasm.

In men, the ejaculation stimulus travels up from the groin via the pudendal nerve to the spinal cord. Once the threshold level of nerve stimulation is reached, nerve impulses automatically flow to the ejaculatory tubes called the vas deferens, to the seminal vesicles, and to the smooth muscles of the prostate gland. This results in ejaculatory fluid going into the pelvic part of the urine tube called the urethra. A reflex closure of the bladder neck prevents ejaculate from going back up into the bladder. Automatic and rhythmic contraction of the perineal muscles and the urethral bulb produces an enjoyable "explosion" of ejaculate out of the urethra.

In women, orgasm is also a genital reflex. Nerve sensations go into the sacral cord, and when the stimuli spills over the threshold level, nerve impulses travel into ovaries, fallopian tubes, vaginal and pubococcygeal muscles, and the uterus. Automatic rhythmic contractions result. During the process, the brain helps the contractions through the release of the amino acid oxytocin, which helps facilitate muscle contractions during sex as well as during childbirth. The release of oxytocin is more important than just for muscle contractions. It rises dramatically in men and women during foreplay and intercourse, increasing sensitivity to the skin and the sexual organs.

Side 7: Sexual Fulfillment and Bliss

How do love, sexual pleasure, and fulfillment relate? Most men do not reach the level of "fulfillment" with sexual activity that women do. The main reason is that men release less oxytocin, which also promotes bonding. This is sometimes called the "touchy, feely" hormone because its levels rise not only during sex but during simple cuddling. It synergizes with estrogen but is antagonized by testosterone.

Oxytocin is the "glue" that bonds a woman to her child. Animal studies show that when oxytocin levels are artificially depressed, a mother will no longer touch her offspring. A low oxytocin level may be a factor in the behavior of women that we periodically read about in newspapers who abandon their newborns.

Because of their comparatively high levels of oxytocin, most women want to be held after an orgasm, whereas men may feel refreshed or exhausted after sexual ejaculation and either want to go to sleep or go on to the next task at hand—work, eat, change the oil in the station wagon. Men's higher levels of free-testosterone levels negate the effects of oxytocin. That's why older men, who have lower free-testosterone levels, are more likely to be warm and cuddly after sex than their younger counterparts.

The strongest T-boosters will have the greatest anti-estrogenic effects. The potent 4-adiol, being the most androgenic, antagonizes
the effects of oxytocin the most. The weakest T-booster, 5-adiol,
probably has the least impact on oxytocin and may even synergize
with it since it is partly estrogenic in its action.

What is sexual bliss? If sexual fulfillment is the physical manifesta-
tion of love, think of sexual bliss as the intellectual and emotional
component. It is a symphonic combination of orgasmic physical sensations that play in concert with a complex mix of brain chemical
messengers, including serotonin, phenylethylamine (PEA), dopamine, and acetylcholine.

Sexual bliss has a spiritual side. Yoga teachers have always told
me to think of orgasm as the equivalent of the total balance of the
physical energy centers of the body called the "chakras." When they
are aligned and your mind is free of all conflict, then you can feel
the cosmic energy called bliss. Yogic bliss and sexual bliss have a lot
in common, both energetically and biochemically speaking. Physiologically, two chemical pathways—dopamine and PEA— are especially important in the feeling of warmth and exhilaration
characteristic of sexual bliss. Interestingly, sexual addiction and
"lovesickness" also share these chemical pathways but in different
ratios. Indeed, lovesickness is really nothing more than a sharp and
sudden decline in dopamine and PEA. When you are deeply in love
and are used to having these chemicals at an elevated level, a rejec-
tion by a lover can send their levels into a tailspin. Watch out! You
might experience a feeling that is the biochemical equivalent of
coming down from a "crack" drug high—irritability, depression,
weepiness, and poor sleep.

People react differently to lovesickness. Some stuff their faces
with chocolate, which is loaded with PEA. Others immediately begin searching, sometimes desperately, for a new lover to "cure"
them. Medically, if a person is lovesick and anxious, then a PEA-like
antidepressant drug such as Wellbutrin might help while the brain
readjusts to the precipitous drop from the former chemical high. In
severe cases I have resorted to prescribing the use of antidepressant
medications to restore some of the chemical messengers responsible
for lovesickness.

From a cold, hard, reductionist way of looking at it, love, or sexual fulfillment and bliss, is simply a triangular biochemical relation-

ship. On one side there is oxytocin for bonding; on a second side, dopamine and PEA for the physical high; and on the third side, serotonin for the warm and fuzzy. Too much of side two, and you could become sexually obsessive or reckless. Too much of side one or two, and you can become "too blissed"—so touchy-feely that you become compulsively possessive or weepy and physically slow and listless.

As you age and your relationship matures, there will be less of the physical high because dopamine and PEA levels go down. The more spiritual and emotional aspects of fulfillment and bliss—the bonding part of the relationship —will remain intact and may even grow.

Side 8: Sexual Bonding — Love and Marriage

Many women and men rush into marriage because they find someone who can stimulate them to an intense sexual high. There is, in fact, a hormonal surge that occurs with new lovers that is comparable to a drug-induced state. Sooner or later the hormone levels do come down, and quite suddenly Mr. or Ms. Right can look terribly ordinary in the light of everyday hormone levels.

It has been theorized that divorce and adultery are so rampant in our contemporary society (50 percent of all marriages end in divorce, and as many 70 percent of spouses admit to at least one extramarital affair) because we're constantly looking for that biochemical honeymoon feeling. A new lover can give you what a longtime partner cannot—a hormonal surge, however temporary it might be. That is probably why the divorce rate of second marriages is no better than that of first marriages. Looking for greener pastures, it turns out that they are the exact same hue. However, if there is a solid and balanced emotional relationship that bonds together the biochemicals of the love triangle, then marriage can survive and prosper.

There are two essential bonding modes: the female track primarily driven by estrogen synergizing with oxytocin, and the male track of testosterones in association with vasopressin.

Like oxytocin, vasopressin is a hormone secreted by the posterior pituitary gland. It helps men be monogamous and stay with a relationship and work it out. It has been shown in animal studies that vasopressin is the hormone that makes males pursue females and then become territorial about them. Vasopressin improves cognition and is considered the "sensible" hormone. Its levels are increased by testosterone and estrogen; when testosterone decreases, so does vasopressin.

T-boosters, then, can indirectly elevate vasopressin through their effect on testosterone. By using T-boosters correctly, we can even influence that most intangible aspect of the Sexual Octagon: commitment or bonding.

Take It Home

The research on how sex hormones affect peripheral tissues—muscles, bones, skin, bladder, urethra, prostate—is clear. The sex hormones ultimately bind into the chromatin—DNA material in the nucleus of a cell. From this process, signals are generated to produce specific proteins. You see the effects on muscle, bone, skin, and other organs that contain sex steroid receptors.

The effect of T-boosters on brain tissue is more subtle because of the functional complexity of the brain tissue and its varied anatomy. The receptors for the sex hormones (estrogens, androgens, and the progesterone family of sex hormones) have been identified in the brain, but because human sexuality itself is multifaceted, exactly how T-boosters work is less clear. Which comes first, sexual interest, sexual arousal, or sexual function? Even if one could find the answer, it would most likely be different for each sex.

We do know conclusively that free testosterone is the sexual energy that drives the engine in our Sexual Octagon model. Like the search engines on the Internet, it allows you to explore many different realms. In our case it is the realms of passion, sexual expression, fantasy cravings, lust, love, and bonding. Without the sexual energy fuel called free testosterone, the biochemical love triangle is hard to maintain.

While men and women manifest human sexuality differently, T-boosters are effective in modulating and influencing sexual interest in both sexes.

~ 7 ~

Super T Sexual Cocktails

Because human sexuality is so complex, almost all of us at some point in our lives will have difficulty in one of the areas described in the last chapter—interest, arousal, and function. With age, declining free-testosterone levels—the fuel that runs the sexual engines in both sexes—increases the likelihood of some type of sexual dysfunction. All women fifty-five or older are in menopause and completely lack free testosterone without intervention. By age fifty at least a quarter of all men experience an abnormal decline in testosterone levels.

Our modern environment seems to wage war against healthy sexuality. We discussed earlier how stress can increase cortisol, which, in turn, decreases free-testosterone levels. Oral birth control can depress free-testosterone levels in women. But there is new evidence of a much more insidious effect. The widespread use of animal hormones, given to livestock for growth, has dramatically increased our exposure to man-made estrogenic and anti-androgenic (anti-testosterone) compounds. The use of potent diethylstilbestrol (DES), once an industry standard, has been stopped. But there are reports that xerolone, another estrogen, is still being used to enhance meat production. Many of these same anti-testosterone compounds are found in herbicides and pesticides.

Couple this with diets that are low in fiber and lack whole grains and fresh fruits and vegetables, and you have a recipe for estrogen overload. It is any wonder there is an increased amount of prostate, breast, and other cancers, as well as low sperm counts, in Western society? In fact, J. Wilson, M.D., reported at the 1998 annual Endocrine Society meeting that in the 1940s routine autopsies showed that about 4 percent of men had breast tissue growth. In the 1990s that number had risen to 20 percent, a fivefold increase.

In this chapter we'll learn how T-booster supplements in various combinations provide a safe and effective antidote to the factors that conspire to upset the delicate balance of sexual hormones. These "sexual cocktails" are customized to fit your individual profile and, best of all, are composed of T-boosters and other supplements that are available over the counter. The cocktails can also be modified to include the prescription drug Viagra if needed.

T-Boosters and Sexual Pleasure

What role does testosterone play in the sexual desire–pleasure equation? It sets the tone and mood for sex by activating four different brain centers. One male brain center involved is the visual aspect of "lust." After taking a Category 1 T-booster, my male patients report noticing sexual nuances and erotic physical features of their sex partners that they had overlooked before.

Two of the brain centers that can be "turned on" with T-boosters are the preoptic and the anterior hypothalamic areas located at the base of the brain. After a T-booster hits one of these sensitive brain areas, the simplest stimuli—a whiff of perfume, for example—can elicit the most erotic thoughts.

Let me share a personal experience: One hour after taking a T-booster, my mind began to wander into sexual fantasies. This was surprising because at that time I was concentrating intensely on cold scientific data. The rest of the day became an erotic voyage in a way that I had not experienced since my teenage years.

Yin-Yang Sexual Modality

While everyone's sexual profile is somewhat individual, biochemically speaking we tend to fall into two dimensions. The first, of course, is gender. The second is what I call yin-estrogen and yang-testosterone modes. These modes are not gender specific. Rather, they indicate the nature of the hormonal ratios.

The ancient Chinese concept of yin and yang was essentially an observation that everything in nature appears to be grouped into pairs of mutually dependent opposites, each of which gives meaning to the other. Thus, "up" has no meaning without "down," or "night" without "day." The same is true for the two primary sex hormones, testosterone and estrogen. They need each other to complete healthy, normal human sexuality.

The questionnaires below will help you decide which of the two primal sexual modes you are in and how to use that insight as a foundation to build your sexual cocktails. First, depending on your gender, you will answer either the male or the female questionnaire. Upon completing the questionnaire you will be directed to one of two modes: the Yin-E(-strogen) or Yang-T(-estosterone). Again, this has nothing to do with conventional ideas of masculine or feminine. Some of my male patients who are hulking bodybuilders are in a Yin-E mode—that is, their hormonal balance is too estrogen rich. But you'd never know that by their appearance or their handshake.

The next step is to find the sexual cocktail that matches your score. Female cocktails and modes will be more variable than a male's because of the sex hormone changes during the menstrual cycle, pregnancy, perimenopause, the menopausal transition (the last five years before the cessation of menstruation), and menopause.

After you have determined your sexual mode, review the modifications to see if they fit your individual profile based on factors such as age, state of health, use of medicines, and the prior or current use of the T-booster described in Chapters 4 and 5 for fat loss and muscle gain. Instructions are given to modify the cocktails accordingly.

The chapter concludes with the Y (yin-yang) files—sexual case histories from my practice that should shed additional light on which sex cocktail is best for you. Keep in mind that there is no such thing as an absolutely guaranteed cocktail that works all the time. I am presenting some general guidelines on how to build them, and individual responses to them will vary. Persons who are generally very sensitive to the environment and have multiple allergies and sensitivities to supplements or medicines should always proceed with caution. They should reduce even further the lowest recommended amounts of the T-boosters and any augmenting supplements given in the sexual cocktails.

Precautions Before Taking Any T Booster Sexual Cocktail

It is important that you read this before taking any T-booster sexual cocktail:

1. ALWAYS start with the *lowest* suggested range of doses. Everyone has a different genetic makeup and metabolizes drugs and supplements differently.

2. DO NOT use any of the pro-sexual formulations if you are in poor health, are out of shape physically, and/or have a serious medical condition. DO NOT use these formulations if you have had a heart attack. If you are out of shape or have heart problems, consult your doctor and have a stress EKG to make sure your heart and body can handle the physical demands of good sex. Exercise of most types increases the chance of a heart attack by two-and-a-half-fold.

3. ALWAYS consult your personal physician before launching into any supplement program that you have not used before. If your physician is not familiar with the biochemistry and actions of T-boosters, buy him or her a copy of this book.

4. If you are on any hormone supplements now, stop using them for four to six weeks to eliminate them from your system before taking a T-booster supplement regimen. These include DHEA, pregnenolone, melatonin, and "underground" steroids as well as any current T-boosters you might be taking. If you are on medically prescribed hormones, including estrogen, progesterone, birth control pills, and testosterone, continue taking them and consult with your doctor.

5. If you have been medically diagnosed with any of the following conditions or are at high risk of developing one of them, do not take T-boosters without first consulting your physician: polycystic ovarian disease, hirsutism (masculinization syndrome of females), gynecomastia (breast growth in men), or other hormonal disorders.

6. Do not use any of the Category 2 T-boosters—the nor-testosterone types—for pro-sexual formulations. They don't make the natural testosterone you need for sexual effect. The only reason to use the nor-testosterone boosters is for muscle gain and fat loss.

Male Questionnaire

Circle the **T** or the **E** at the end of each question if the question applies to your personal condition. Only circle the **T** or **E** if it applies.

1. Do you have low sexual interest or a low sex drive? **E**
2. Do you prefer one-night stands to an ongoing sexual relationship? **T**
3. Are you bloated or feel bloated a lot of the time? **E**
4. Do you have an unusual degree of sugar and carbohydrate cravings? **E**
5. Have you recently gained weight that is mostly from fat rather than muscle? **E**
6. Are you getting excessively aggressive—which is out of character for you? **T**
7. Would you rather be cuddled by someone than have an orgasm by yourself or with someone? **E**
8. Do you feel a need for orgasm any way you can get it, more than a need for "lovemaking"? **T**
9. Do you feel excessively sluggish? **E**
10. Is your skin getting excessively oily, with more acne than usual? **T**
11. Is your body odor getting more pungent than usual? **T**
12. Are you considered too cocky and overconfident by your peers? **T**
13. Are you always horny and have sex on your mind? **T**
14. Are your muscles getting really big without your taking any anabolic hormones or doing a lot of weight training? **T**
15. Does your skin flush or get red-pink very easily? **E**
16. Does being receptive to intercourse dominate your need for orgasm? **E**
17. Do you have an excessive amount of sexual desire? **T**
18. Do you have any medically diagnosed problems that are immune problems, such as the autoimmune disorders (systemic lupus erythematosis [SLE], multiple sclerosis, rheumatoid arthritis)? **E**
19. Do you tend to be a sexual athlete rather than a "lover"? **T**

20. Are your muscles getting flabby despite working out and eating right? **E**
21. Are you a heavy meat eater? **T**
22. Are you irritable in a weepy kind of way? **E**
23. Do you need to masturbate more than once a day and prefer masturbation to sexual intercourse? **T**
24. Are you rapidly and prematurely losing your hair? **T**
25. Have you noted your testicles are getting smaller? **E**
26. Do you have to work harder than your peers to gain muscle in the gym despite all the right foods or supplements and training? **E**
27. Is your body odor losing its normal pungent smell? **E**
28. Has your sexual interest declined? **E**
29. Is your waist size bulging over your belt line? **E**
30. Have you recently been told you are overly aggressive? **T**
31. Are you having fewer erections in the mornings when you first wake up? **E**
32. Have you noted decreased facial hair or the need to shave less often? **E**

Male Scores

Add up the total number of **T**'s circled. Then add up the total number of **E**'s circled. Which of the following applies to you?

1. If your **T** score is equal to your **E** score or they are within 2 of each other, you have a balanced yin-yang sexual mode.
2. If your **T** score exceeds your **E** score by 3, you have a moderate yang sexual mode.
3. If your **T** score is 4 or more than your **E** score, you have a high yang sexual mode.
4. If your **E** score is more than your **T** score by 3, you have a moderate yin sexual mode.
5. If your **E** score is 4 or more than your **T** score, you have a high yin sexual mode.

The scores correspond with the Super T cocktails below. The cocktails are divided into two types: those with Viagra and those without. Medically, most men do not need Viagra. If you do not have a problem with getting and maintaining an erection, then you are wasting your money on Viagra. Try the cocktails in the first section. That said, I know enough about human nature that many of you who don't need Viagra will try it anyway. So please, if you do take the T-booster cocktails with Viagra, please read the precautions provided in that section.

Men: Super T Cocktails (Without Viagra)

Moderate Yin Sexual Mode

Problem: moderate excess estrogenic effect, low testosterone level. Most men in this mode feel sluggish, bloated, emotional, and even depressed. They also have a decreased sexual appetite and an inability to lose weight.

Solution: This is a two-part program. Part A helps build energy reserves and should be initiated three to five days before a planned session of lovemaking. Part B has specific recommendations for the day of lovemaking.

Part A (Three to Five Days)

1. Take 2.5 to 5 milligrams of NADH (nicotinamide adenine dinucleotide, available over the counter) in the morning with water one hour before breakfast.

•➤*Note:* A trade name of NADH is Enanda. It must come in a sealed blister pack to be the real stuff.

2. Make sure you're taking B vitamins at levels recommended in Antiaging Cocktail (see page 77).
3. Experiment with 500 to 1,000 milligrams of L-tyrosine, two to three times daily, to see if your mood improves and your energy increases. Do not take at the same time as NADH; separate by four to six hours.

•➤*Caution:* Avoid L-tyrosine if you have heart problems, high blood pressure, or are an anxious person.

4. Experiment with 400 to 800 milligrams of the yohimbé standardized extract, one to three times daily. Use the "stamp test"
described in the last chapter to test its effectiveness.

•→ *Caution:* Some people get anxious and feel hot with yohimbé;
it may elevate heart rate and blood pressure. If so, cut back on
the dose.

5. Every other day take 50 to 100 milligrams of 4-adiol, one to
two times daily.

Part B (Lovemaking Day)

Use only the agents that caused you no discomfort in Part A. Below
is a sample program.

1. NADH in the morning before breakfast
2. 100 milligrams of 4-adiol or 50 milligrams of adiol plus 50 milligrams of adione in the morning with breakfast
3. One hour before sex, 100 milligrams of adione with or without 400 to 800 milligrams of yohimbé standardized extract.

High Yin Sexual Mode

The program above can be modified slightly to accommodate men
with a high yin score.

Part A

1. Use the program for a minimum of four days.
2. Try all the supplements in the moderate program at the mid
to high ranges.
3. Add 1,000 to 1,500 milligrams of acetyl L-carnitine to the 5-
milligram NADH dose in the morning.
4. Use 100 milligrams of 4-adiol two or three times daily for at
least three days.
5. Avoid exhaustive exercise.

6. Add 60 milligrams of gingko biloba three times daily for at least three days.

Part B (Lovemaking Day)

1. 2.5 to 5 milligrams of NADH in the morning
2. 500 to 1,000 milligrams of L-tyrosine in the late afternoon, taken on an empty stomach
3. Gingko biloba: 60 milligrams in the morning, 60 milligrams in the afternoon, and 120 milligrams two hours before sex
4. 100 milligrams of 4-adiol in the morning with breakfast, 50 milligrams of 4-adiol plus 50 milligrams of adione with lunch, and 100 milligrams of adione one hour before sex, along with your yohimbine. Add 4 to 8 grams of L-arginine on an empty stomach thirty to forty-five minutes before sex.

Moderate Yang Sexual Mode

Problem: Too orgasm-driven, too aggressive, "amped-up." Inability to have sex in a loving way.
Solution: This is a two-part program. Part A should be initiated three to five days before a planned session of lovemaking. Part B has specific recommendations for the day of lovemaking.

Part A (Three to Five Days)

1. Decrease red meat in your diet and concentrate on fruits and vegetable proteins.
2. Increase calcium intake to 500 to 1,000 milligrams and magnesium intake to 500 to 800 milligrams.
3. Take standardized kava kava two or three times a day.
4. Try 5-hydroxytryptophan (5-HTP) at 50 to 150 milligrams to relax.
5. Take 50 milligrams of nor-adione or nor-4-adiol in the morning and the afternoon for at least three days in a row.
6. Exercise with long cardiovascular workouts. (See Appendix 3)

Part B (Lovemaking Day)

1. Take 50 milligrams of nor-adione and 50 milligrams of nor-4-adiol with breakfast and lunch. One hour before sex, take 50 to 100 milligrams of nor-4-adiol.
2. Increase your morning cardiovascular workout.
3. Take two or three capsules of standardized kava kava extract and 50 to 100 milligrams of 5-HTP one hour before sex.

High Yang Sexual Mode

The moderate yang program above can be modified slightly to accommodate men with a high yang score.

Parts A and B

Increase all the above recommendations for the moderate yang sexual mode to the higher dose and frequency for Part A and Part B programs. In addition, modify Part B as follows:

1. Do a very intense cardiovascular workout in the morning and before sex.
2. Take 100 milligrams of nor-4-adiol with breakfast, again at lunch, and again one hour before sex.
3. Take 100 to 200 milligrams of 5-HTP one hour before sex, along with a larger dose of kava kava—but not so much that it will make you sleep.

The Problem with Viagra

Since March 1998, when Viagra was first released to the public, more than 50 million diamond-shaped blue tablets have been consumed. The question is: by whom? Since then insurance companies have tightened their eligibility restrictions because it became apparent that many of those 50 million pills consumed were not used by impotent men with medically defined erectile dysfunction.

A sizable portion of Viagra sales are to young men who find themselves impotent because of lifestyle choices—for example, indulging in too much alcohol, tobacco, and fatty foods. They do not need Viagra; they need to change their lifestyles. They could have excellent natural sex if they cleaned up their acts. The fact is that most young men under thirty-five don't need Viagra. Many of those who think they need it report surpassingly disappointing results. One of my patients reported that Viagra sex for him was an impersonal experience, like watching someone else making love. He obtained an erection, but there was no emotionality. Erections have little to do with testosterone or with sexual craving, desire, or emotional fulfillment.

As a modern medical culture, we are now witnesses to a schizophrenic sexual phenomenon—the non-sex-hormone mediated sexual experience. Viagra has created a disassociation between erections and lust. A "hard-on" is achieved simply by popping a pill and indulging in minimal erotic stimulation.

T-boosters more closely mimic the way the body produces testosterone than any medically prescribed testosterone product. Nocturnal and morning erections can occur despite the return to baseline of testosterone blood levels three to four hours after T-booster ingestion. However, T-boosters will not produce the erection-on-command effect of Viagra.

One of the advantages of combining T-boosters and Viagra at night is to take advantage of the residual erectile effect that occurs in the morning. The biochemically induced nighttime sex will help facilitate the naturally occurring erections the following morning. Plan your schedule so that you can have great morning sex in addition to your potent evening sexual experience.

Precautions and Guidelines for Viagra

These rules must be followed to ensure that you have a safe and effective T-booster/Viagra sexual experience. Use them in addition to the precautions presented earlier in the chapter.

1. Do not use Viagra with the following medications: nitroglycerin-containing compounds such as Nitro-Bid and Nitrostat; isosorbide mononitrates such as Imdur Isosorbide; isosorbide

dinitrates such as Dilatrate-SR and Isordil; and other nitrate-containing drugs or "poppers"—amyl nitrate.

2. Do not use Viagra with any prescription yohimbine or supplements containing yohimbine or yohimbé. In some sensitive men it can trigger a condition called priapism, a prolonged painful erection lasting for more than three hours. *It is a medical emergency. If not treated, irreversible damage to the penis may occur.* If priapism does occur, go to the emergency room. The standard treatment is to inject vasoconstricting medicines into the penis and remove the trapped blood from the penis by needle extraction. Oral medications that can help by causing a constriction of blood vessels include ephedrine, Sudafed (pseudoephedrine), and caffeine. However, avoid taking these if you have high blood pressure or an irregular heartbeat.

3. Frail, sickly, or deconditioned individuals should not use any of these formulations with Viagra *at all*. Persons with heart disease or on multiple medications should refrain from the use of Viagra.

Follow these general rules for taking Viagra:

- Take 25 to 100 milligrams before sex. You can cut a 100-milligram tablet into quarters or halves to save money (even though the manufacturer does not recommend it).
- It is best taken on an empty stomach, or after a light non-fatty, mainly carbohydrate meal (pasta and a salad, for example), or three to four hours after a heavy meal. Fatty meals delay absorption and the onset and potency of Viagra. (The T-boosters supplement in the Sexual Cocktails are less affected by food.)
- If you want a quicker onset of action, grind up the Viagra and put it into a shot of fruit juice. The onset of action is noted by flushing and then an erection within thirty minutes as opposed to the usual hour.

Men: Super T Cocktails (with Viagra)

Find the cocktail below that corresponds to your male questionnaire score.

Balanced Yin-Yang Sexual Mode

You do not have to take any special measures. To help achieve erection, use intermittently 50 to 100 milligrams of adione, one to two hours before sex or, in combination with Viagra, one hour before sex.

Moderate Yang Sexual Mode

Use 50 to 100 milligrams of nor-adione or nor-4-adiol two to three hours before taking Viagra. Androstenedione will help suppress your tendency toward excesses of yang sexual mode energy before you engage in sex. The overall effect of the cocktail will be to increase libido while promoting a more profound sexual experience.

High Yang Sexual Mode

Use the T-boosters with the lower libido potencies, such as nor-4-adiol (50 to 100 milligrams) or no T-boosters at all. You definitely should not use the potent 4-adiol, which could exacerbate your excessive yang energy. Take Viagra one hour before sex. Take T-boosters once or twice daily for one day before sex and two to three hours before sex. Follow the guidelines in Chapter 8 to modify your lifestyle, diet, and exercise to decrease the effects of your testosterone overload.

Moderate Yin Sexual Mode

Take Viagra one hour before sex. To charge up your yang energy, take 50 to 100 milligrams of androstenedione, or in combination with 50 to 100 milligrams of 4-adiol, once or twice daily for one to three days before sex. Also take 50 to 100 milligrams of adione or 4-adiol one to two hours before sex. Since you have some excess estrogen, avoid 5-adiol. Follow the guidelines in Chapter 8 on how to deal with excess estrogen.

High Yin Sexual Mode

You appear to be extremely testosterone deficient or have extreme excess estrogen. Use only Category 1 T-boosters. Males with high yin scores need a lot of the libido T-boosters 4-adiol or adione. You can try to modify your sexual mode by taking 50 to 100 milligrams of 4-adiol, adione, or a combination of both twice a day for three days to build up sexual interest before sex, and then 100 milligrams with Viagra one hour before sex. You can also modify your sexual mode by adding more monosaturated fats from oils such as olive, almond, or macadamia nut, and cruciferous vegetables to help with elimination of excess yin estrogens from your body. Follow the guidelines in Chapter 8 on increasing your testosterone levels.

Cocktail Modifications for Viagra Due to Age or Lifestyle

Older men (fifty-five to sixty-five) should start with 25 to 50 milligrams of Viagra and increase the dose slowly if there is no effect. The higher the dose, the greater the chance of side effects, including visual sensitivity to bright lights, seeing a blue to yellow haze around lights, upset stomach, headache, stuffy nose, or dizziness.

Smokers, diabetics, and hypersensitive and anxious men have poorer penile circulation and more problems with erections. These men may need Viagra doses at the higher end, but in the beginning they should always start with no more than 50 milligrams.

Men: Super Sexual Cocktail

Healthy men forty-five to fifty-five years old might want to consider taking this advanced Sexual Cocktail formula. Remember, there are individual responses to all dosages given in this book. Start at the low range and monitor the effect. If necessary, increase the dosage slowly but never exceed the upper range. Do not use with any mind-altering prescription drugs, including antidepressants, or with any similar nonprescription supplements.

Follow these steps:

1. Four to six hours before sex, take 2.5 to 5 milligrams of NADH supplement with water on an empty stomach. If you feel too "amped up" or are naturally anxious, dampen the effect with some kava.

2. Take 100 to 200 milligrams of 4-adiol or adione one hour before sex.

3. Add 50 to 100 milligrams of Viagra. Do not eat heavily if using Viagra.

Most likely there will be some residual erectile effect the next day, so schedule your time for sex accordingly. Make sure you are well rested. Avoid excessive alcohol and all other drugs. (One to two glasses of wine or beer is fine.)

Female Questionnaire

Circle the **T** or the **E** at the end of each question if the question applies to your personal condition. Only circle the **T** or **E** if it applies.

•→*Note:* Some answers have multiple **T**'s or **E**'s, and each one should be counted separately. For example, "**E E**" equals two.

1. Do you have low sexual interest or a low sex drive? **E**
2. Do you prefer one-night stands to an ongoing sexual relationship? **T**
3. Are you bloated or feel bloated a lot of the time? **E**
4. Do you have an unusual degree of sugar and carbo-starch cravings? **E**
5. Is your skin getting rough or coarse for no reason? **T**
6. Have you recently gained weight that is mostly from fat rather than muscle? **E**
7. Are you getting excessively aggressive—which is out of character for you? **T**
8. Would you rather be cuddled by someone than have an orgasm by yourself or with someone? **E**
9. Do you feel a need for orgasm any way you can get it, more than a need for "lovemaking"? **T**

10. Do you feel excessively sluggish? **E**
11. Is your skin getting excessively oily, with more acne than usual? **T**
12. Is your body odor getting more pungent than usual? **T**
13. Has your waist size expanded excessively? **E**
14. Are you considered too cocky or overconfident by your peers? **T**
15. Are you always horny and have sex on your mind? **T**
16. Are your muscles getting really big without your taking any anabolic hormones or doing a lot of weight training? **T**
17. Does your skin flush or get red-pink very easily? **E**
18. Does being receptive to intercourse dominate your need for orgasm? **E**
19. Do you have an excessive amount of sexual desire? **T**
20. Do you have any medically diagnosed autoimmune disorders such as systemic lupus erythematosis (SLE), multiple sclerosis, rheumatoid arthritis, or fibromyalgia? **E**
21. Would you rather be a sexual athlete than a "lover"? **T**
22. Are your muscles getting flabby despite working out and eating right? **E**
23. Are you a heavy meat eater? **T**
24. Are you irritable in a weepy kind of way? **E**
25. Do you need to masturbate more than once a day and prefer masturbation to sexual intercourse? **T**
26. Are you rapidly and prematurely losing your hair, or is it thinning? **T**
27. Do you have to work harder than your peers to gain muscle in the gym despite all the right foods or supplements and training? **E**
28. Has your sexual interest declined? **E**
29. Have you noted growth of thick, textured hair similar to hair seen on the male body, not the soft downy type of female hair? Is it located above the upper lip, at the chin, around the breasts or abdomen? **T T T**
30. Do your breasts swell often, more than might be normally expected? **E**
31. Do you often have breast pain more than you might expect from menstrual fluctuations or estrogen replacement? **E E**
32. Is your voice getting unusually deeper? **T**

33. Do you have excessive amounts of vaginal lubrication even when not sexually aroused? **E E**
34. Are you losing hair in the pattern normally known as male pattern at the temples and at the crown of the head? **T T**

Female Scores

Add up the total number of **T**'s circled. Then add up the total number of **E**'s circled. Which of the following applies to you?

1. If your **T** score is equal to your **E** score or they are within 2 of each other, you have a balanced yin-yang sexual mode.
2. If your **E** score exceeds your **T** score by 3, you have a moderate yin sexual mode.
3. If your **E** score is 4 or more than your **T** score, you have a high yin sexual mode.
4. If your **T** score exceeds your **E** score by 3, you have a moderate yang sexual mode.
5. If your **T** score is 4 or more than your **E** score, you have a high yang sexual mode.

Find below the Super T cocktail that corresponds with your sexual mode score.

Women and Viagra

You will note that none of the following formulations for women's cocktails contain Viagra. There are no definitive studies on the effects of Viagra on women, although research is under way in Europe and elsewhere on postmenopausal women. Until these results are known, it is best for women not to use it.

Viagra was designed for the male performance system, which is dependent on getting blood into and staying inside the penis. However, a woman's arousal system also signals blood to flow into the sexual regions, involving the labia, clitoris, and vagina, resulting in engorgement, lubrication, and increased sensitivity to touch.

Young women with normal to high estrogen levels who take

Viagra may experience excessive flushing and intense headaches and nasal congestion. Estrogen and Viagra are both blood vessel dilators, so there can be a synergistic effect. Older women who are on estrogen replacement therapy can experience the same effects, and the combination of drugs can potentially precipitate migraine headaches.

So far, early anecdotal clinical reports from my colleagues and my own small clinical trials of 12.5 to 25 milligrams of Viagra doses suggest some positive response to Viagra in older women who are not on estrogen and don't normally easily flush or have hot flashes. There may be some increase of vaginal lubrication and sensitization of the clitoris.

Women: Super T Cocktails

Balanced Yin-Yang Sexual Mode

Your score indicates you have a well-rounded sexuality with no special needs. To enhance your sexual experience, take 10 to 25 milligrams of androstenedione, one to two hours before sex no more than one or two times a week.

Moderate Yin Sexual Mode

Your score indicates that you have a moderate excess of yin (estrogen). Follow all the diet, exercise, and lifestyle modifications in Chapter 8 to balance your yin mode. Begin by taking 10 to 25 milligrams of androstenedione or 4-adiol two hours before sex, two to three times a week or periodically, to increase your sexual interest. Monitor its effectiveness and, if needed, gradually increase to the upper range of dose and frequency.

High Yin Sexual Mode

Your score indicates a high excess of yin (estrogen). Follow the dietary, exercise, and lifestyle modifications in Chapter 8 to decrease yin. Begin by taking 10 to 25 milligrams of androstenedione or 4-

adiol three or four times a week and especially before sex. Follow the guidelines in Chapter 8 to balance excess yin (estrogen) with the phytoestrogens (weak plant estrogens) to modify the potent and unfriendly synthetic estrogens.

Moderate Yang Sexual Mode

Your score indicates an excess of androgens-testosterone. Consult your doctor if it accelerates.

Do not use any T-boosters. Follow the guidelines in Chapter 8 for the yang sexual mode.

High Yang Sexual Mode

Your score indicates that you have an excessively high level of androgens-testosterone. Consult an endocrinologist who specializes in sex hormones. Do not use any T-boosters.

Women: Super Sexual Cocktail

Healthy women forty to fifty-five years old might want to consider taking this advanced Sexual Cocktail formula. Remember, there are individual responses to all dosages given in this book. Start at the low range and monitor the effect. If necessary, increase the dosage slowly but never take more than the upper range. Do not use with any mind-altering prescription, including antidepressants, or with any similar nonprescription supplements.

Follow these steps:

1. Four to six hours before sex, take 2.5 to 5 milligrams of NADH (Enada) supplement. If you feel too "amped up" or are naturally anxious, dampen the effect with some kava kava.
2. Take 25 to 50 milligrams of 4-adiol, one hour before sex.

Most likely there will be a good deal of residual sexual effect the next day, so schedule your lovemaking time accordingly. Make sure you are well rested. Avoid excessive alcohol and all other drugs. (One to two glasses of wine or beer is fine.)

The Y Files

A variety of yin-yang sexual problems can be corrected by a T-booster supplement regimen. The following age-related problems are based on case histories taken from the files of my clinic, the Sports Medicine and Anti-Aging Medical Group in Santa Monica, California.

Women: Ages Twenty to Thirty

During their early twenties, most women are estrogen dominant and therefore "receptively driven" and looking for love and bonding with a partner rather than simply sexual pleasure in relationships. Their high degree of oxytocin helps cement their relationships. When women reach their late twenties, there is a tendency in many to shift toward orgasmic testosterone-driven sex.

Common hormonal sexual problems include low orgasmic drive and estrogen overload swelling, breast tenderness, bloating, decreased muscle mass, and increased weight. This is made worse by birth control pills containing estrogen. The all-progesterone birth control pills are versions of nor-testosterone, as are the Category 2 T-boosters. These oral contraceptives may have anti-estrogen and male effects.

Remedy: An occasional dose (one to two times a month) of low-potency T-boosters such as androstenedione can be helpful. A small dose of 4-adiol may boost sexual desire. It is not unusual for 4-adiol to cause a woman to be a little more aggressive and bold for three to six hours. In addition, adding soy to the diet may decrease estrogen excess and promote hormonal balance.

•➤ *Caution:* These supplements have not been fully studied. Long-term effects are not known, and fertility may be affected.

Men: Ages Twenty to Thirty

Most men in their twenties are performance (testosterone)-driven and focused on orgasm. Many feel they must prove they can make the female respond, so the bedroom becomes a battleground. Men in this age group are often disconnected from the emotional part of sex, which estrogen-dominant females of this age desire.

Women: Ages Thirty to Forty

While women in their twenties are estrogen-driven to a biological peak of sexual receptiveness, by their thirties they are testosterone-driven toward a peak of sexual pleasure and orgasms. At this stage most women become more independent, socially and sexually, and many women are ending relationships started in their twenties. Many start careers and try to be independent of men financially; developing their careers often takes priority over relationships.

These changes in behavior occur because of a changing sex hormone profile. Women become more testosterone-dominated as they grow older. The net effect is a lowering of the estrogen-to-testosterone ratio. As estrogen declines, the testosterone mental effect becomes pronounced. Thus, women in their thirties are more likely to become sexual pleasure seekers than they were in their twenties.

In addition, lower estrogen levels cause an increase in the free active portion of testosterone via a lower level of the protein that clings to the testosterone.

Men: Ages Thirty to Forty

Men's testosterone and estrogen levels start to equalize. At this stage most men begin to wise up about sex and the needs of their sexual partners. They have gotten over the "jackhammer" sexual performance stage of their teens and early twenties and have begun to desire bonding and closeness. As the testosterone dominance of their twenties diminishes, they start to connect sex with their emotions and begin to desire commitment.

Women: Ages Forty to Fifty

By forty, women's testosterone levels begin to bottom out. Most women start to feel the effects of this androgen deficiency, such as less muscle mass or an increase in fat levels and an inability to lose weight. This does not always correlate with a low sex drive. A woman may have low testosterone but have a strong dopamine system that drives her sexually. This usually occurs in women who have low serotonin levels in the brain. Women often like younger men at this stage in their lives.

When women hit the mid-forties, perimenopause often appears. Hormonal, menstrual, and emotional fluctuations occur as the ovaries are declining in their estrogen output. Women often suffer from "hot flashes," and many women have trouble sleeping.

By age fifty, 80 to 90 percent of women are in menopause, and many experience a difficult time with their sex lives.

Men: Ages Forty to Fifty

By this age most men notice a drop in their sex drive, feel tired and less ambitious, and have a decreased capacity for getting and maintaining firm erections. Prostate problems start to manifest with frequent nighttime urination, a decrease in the arc and force of the urinary stream, and an increased difficulty in stopping and starting urination. In addition, their waistlines begin to spread, and they have more trouble building muscle despite proper workouts.

Women: Ages Fifty to Sixty

At age fifty-five, women universally reach menopause and face questions of whether to use hormone replacements and, if so, which types and how. Women at this stage of life often gain weight and develop mood changes. Irritability, fatigue, and depression are common complaints. Decreased sexual interest can be a result of depression and a universally low free-testosterone blood level. Most women notice that everything seems to be working slower, and they may notice a decline in memory. Vaginal atrophy and urinary and lubrication problems are also common.

Men: Ages Fifty to Sixty

At this stage of life in America, most men share the common problems of low energy, weight gain, low sex drive, decreased erectile function, and prostate and heart problems. The old college sports injuries of the back, hips, and knees are prominently felt.

Women: Ages Sixty to Eighty

Weak bones, osteoporosis, and loss of muscle mass and hip fractures are common by this age. The joints ache and creak. Who wants to have sex when your knees, hips, and back hurt? Fortunately, a T-booster regimen can help turn back the symptoms of aging.

Men: Ages Sixty to Eighty

The prostate can be a big problem at this age. Urinary and prostate difficulties or the effects of prostate surgery frequently interfere with sexual function and desire.

Take It Home

All of us likely will have some type of sexual problem at one time or another. T-boosters are a safe and effective remedy for many of these problems. However, different T-boosters can have different effects, so it is important to determine your sexual profile before embarking on a supplement program.

There are two primary dimensions to our sexual profiles: gender and mode, which is either yin-estrogen or yang-testosterone. Healthy sexuality depends on a proper biochemical balance between the two sexual energies, in both men and women.

For men with a sexual performance problem, a T-booster cocktail containing Viagra can be a powerful antidote. Most men under forty do not need and should not take Viagra. The verdict is still out on the effectiveness of Viagra on women.

8

Pro-Sexual Lifestyle Strategies

What is the better marker of good health, a good sex life or a good cardiovascular system? Many studies have shown that persons who maintain sexual interest and are sexually active are in better health overall than those with low sexual interest and who have a low frequency of sexual activity. In fact, sexual activity is a better indicator of longevity than just exercise alone. That is, those who are sexually active are more likely to live longer than those who are not,

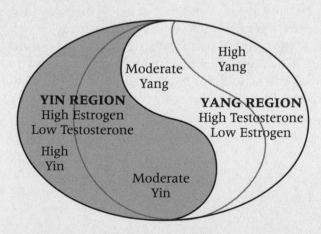

FIGURE 7—*The Yin-Yang of Hormonal Harmony*

even if they are less physically fit than their asexual counterparts, all other things being equal.

This chapter is a guide for creating a lifestyle with a balance between your yin (estrogen-dominant) and yang (testosterone-dominant) sexual modes. Both men and women have estrogen and testosterone. These hormones have identical chemical structures in both genders. The only difference is in the amount and pattern of production and the ratios between them.

Chapter 7 offered T-booster sexual cocktails to help balance your sexual yin and yang, for the purpose of enhancing sexual interest, sexual behavior, and sexual function. This chapter complements the cocktails by outlining long-term strategies to balance hormones with diet, exercise, and lifestyle choices. If your score shows that your yin and yang sexual hormones are balanced and in harmony, you have probably already adopted many of the suggestions in this chapter and have a healthy lifestyle. This chapter, then, is mainly intended for those who scored moderate or high on the yin-yang questionnaire and need some sexual balancing or lifestyle modifications.

The core programs presented below will probably be adequate if you scored in the moderate range. If you scored high in either yin or yang sexual energy, follow the appropriate modifications. Further modifications to the core program are designed for all women.

Yin Lifestyle Strategies: A Testosterone-Boosting / Estrogen-Lowering Program

This program is designed to boost testosterone and limit its conversion to estrogen. Use this program if you scored in the moderate yin sexual mode in Chapter 7. If you have a moderate yin, this core program will probably be adequate for your balancing needs. However, if you scored 5 or above, this program may not be enough; consult the section below for modifications for high yin mode.

The source of the excess yin (moderate estrogen elevation plus low testosterone) could have many origins:

1. Excess intake of estrogens. This includes prescription estrogens in birth control pills or estrogen replacement therapies.
2. Increased substrate. These are substances from which you can make estrogen via increased DHEA and androstenedione production by the adrenal glands, or from excessive or inappropriate supplementation with DHEA or androstenedione, 5-adiol, and other T-boosters.
3. Increase of fat stores. Obesity causes an increase of conversion of testosterone to estrogen by the very active immature fat cells called pre-adipocytes.
4. Decreased capacity to eliminate excess estrogen. This is caused by liver damage from alcohol, drugs, or the use of various medications (see Appendix 2).
5. Low fiber/vegetable intake, especially from cruciferous vegetables such as broccoli, cauliflower, Brussels sprouts, and cabbage.
6. Low soy diet. Soy products can modulate estrogen excesses.
7. Low citrus/vitamin C intake. The exception is grapefruit, which can increase estrogen levels.
8. The wrong type of fats. Generally speaking, a diet high in the omega-6 oils (polyunsaturates) will decrease testosterone.
9. Eating meats containing estrogens. Livestock is frequently given a pro-estrogen hormone called Xerolone.
10. Exposure to, or intake of, anti-androgens/pro-estrogens. These include pesticides, herbicides, and certain medications or oral birth control pills.
11. Aging in men. Older men have increased activity of an enzyme (aromatase) that converts testosterone to estrogen.
12. Uncontrolled stress. Anxiety and depression cause testosterone and sperm level to decrease.
13. Overtraining. This means chronically doing too much exercise, such as a triathlon or marathon, or constantly training hard without enough recovery time.

Diet

A proper balance of all three macronutrients—fats, carbohydrates, and protein—is essential for a proper hormonal balance.

A. Carbohydrates

If you don't consume enough carbohydrates, your body takes this as a sign of stress and lowers your testosterone levels. Most people eat enough carbohydrates in their diets, but if you eat too much meat, fish, and other proteins while neglecting high-carbohydrate foods, you may be causing your testosterone levels to go down.

Carbohydrate-restricted diets such as the high-fat (50 percent), high-protein (40 percent) Atkins diet have become popular recently. These diets can be helpful for losing weight but should be followed for a short time since they will have a negative effect on testosterone levels. This does not mean you should load up on simple carbohydrates such as sugar, pasta, and white bread, but you should make an effort to eat four to six servings of whole grain foods and legumes such as rye or whole wheat bread, buckwheat, oatmeal, beans, peas, lentils, brown rice, and sweet potatoes. You should also have five to ten servings of fruits and vegetables throughout the day.

B. Proteins

A study done at Penn State University showed protein to have a higher negative correlation with testosterone than any other macronutrient. A very high protein diet stimulates enzymes in the liver to break down both testosterone and estrogen, and eliminate them from the body. For young men and women this could accelerate their yin sexual mode. In menopausal women and older men this could accelerate bone loss.

The type of protein in your diet will also affect your testosterone levels. I believe a good balance of protein in your diet for both testosterone maximization and muscle maintenance is roughly two-thirds of a gram of protein per pound of body weight per day. This would be 100 grams (15 ounces of lean chicken, turkey, fish, low-fat cheese, or twenty-five egg whites) for a 150-pound person, and 67 grams (about 9 ounces) for a 100-pound person.

The best sources of protein for boosting testosterone are meat, fish, egg whites (albumin), and milk. If you have health risks associated with too much fat, eat lean sources such as skinless chicken breasts, egg whites, whey protein, or casein proteins derived from milk.

You can also buy supplement powders that contain mixtures of proteins derived from egg whites and milk. If you are on a tight budget, use egg whites and nonfat dry milk as your protein sources. Eat non-oily fish if calories are a big concern, or fish such as salmon, Chilean sea bass, sardines, and swordfish (which contain healthy oils), but in smaller portions.

Eating all your daily protein at one time is a waste of effort and money. Your body assimilates protein best when it is eaten in small, frequent quantities, so it's best to get your protein in doses of 20 to 40 grams, three to six times daily. How much protein you need depends on your body weight. See Appendix 1, Table 5, to help you plan your meals.

C. Fats

Most people concerned with their health make a conscious effort to eliminate fat from their diets. However, a diet too low in fat will cause testosterone levels to drop significantly. The Penn State study found certain types of fat highly and positively correlated with testosterone levels. They were saturated fats and monounsaturated fatty acids (MUFAs), the latter found in high levels in olive oil, canola oil, avocado oil, macadamia nuts, and almonds.

It is true that diets high in saturated (animal) fats have been linked to high cholesterol levels and heart disease. However, MUFAs can lower cholesterol levels, thus lowering the risk of heart disease. Diets high in MUFAs have been linked to lower LDL (bad) cholesterol levels and higher HDL (good) cholesterol and testosterone levels.

Eat moderate amounts of healthy sources of MUFAs; they provide energy, boost testosterone levels, satisfy hunger, and may protect against heart disease. Aim to have roughly 30 percent of your calories from fat.

Below is a ranking of some oils by their percentage of MUFAs. Use this information when deciding which oils to consume. The monounsaturated oils are somewhat heat stable and can be used for cooking. As a general rule, don't burn cooking oil. The worst oils to cook with or eat are the unstable polyunsaturates such as corn, soybean, sunflower, and safflower. (See Table 1, item 4, in Appendix 1.)

Oil	Percentage of MUFA
Virgin Olive	68
Canola	57
Rice Bran	48
Sesame	45
Soybean	32
Flaxseed	22

YIN (HIGH SCORE) SAMPLE MEAL PLAN

BREAKFAST

5 to 10 egg whites scrambled with 2 to 4 teaspoons of canola oil; occasionally 1 yolk may be added

1 to 2 pieces of toast with 1 to 2 tablespoons of peanut butter

1 to 2 pieces of fruit

LUNCH

1 to 2 cups of vegetable soup (clear broth; no creams)

1 to 2 grilled chicken breast halves

1 to 2 cups of vegetables

1/2 to 1 cup of cooked pasta with marinara sauce, 1 tablespoon of olive oil, and a choice of spices (turmeric, cayenne pepper, and garlic are good choices)

DINNER

1 to 2 cups of green salad with lots of colorful vegetables with 1 to 2 tablespoons of low-fat olive oil–based dressing

3 to 6 ounces of grilled fish of your choice

1/2 to 1 cup of wild or brown rice blended with 2 to 4 teaspoons of olive or canola oil with your choice of sauce or seasonings

1 to 2 cups of steamed green and yellow vegetables

1 to 2 cups of fresh or thawed frozen raspberries

SNACK

2 to 4 sticks of low-fat or nonfat string cheese

1 to 2 pieces of fruit

Diet Modifications for High LDL Cholesterol

If your cholesterol levels are too high, you may want to switch from animal protein sources to primarily vegetable protein sources. The best overall source is the whole soybean, which is served as "edamame" in Japanese restaurants or available frozen in health food or Japanese markets. Roasted whole soybeans (soy nuts) taste like peanuts but are higher in protein and lower in fat. Do not eat too many because they are relatively high in PUFAs (polyunsaturated fats) and, during roasting, a lot of PUFA might become toxic.

Personally, I also like to boil batches of dry whole soybeans (after soaking them in water overnight) or use canned black soybeans. I add them to salads and soups, and eat them as side dishes. If you don't like the taste of soy products such as tofu, soy milk, and tempeh, there are many soy products that taste like meat after the addition of a few spices. You can make a dynamite chili from soybean-textured vegetable protein (TVP) and pinto beans. There are also good-tasting soy protein drinks and bars (see Appendix 1, Table 2).

If you are lifting weights to build muscle, you may also want to add a soy-whey protein supplement to your diet. Whey protein is a high-quality source of animal protein that has many health benefits, and unlike other animal proteins, it probably will not cause your cholesterol levels to go up.

By switching to vegetable sources of protein, your testosterone levels will not be as high as they would be if you relied primarily on animal protein sources. But as long as you are consuming a balanced amount of MUFAs and carbohydrates, you will still have healthy testosterone levels.

Diet Modifications for Fat Loss and Muscle Gain

If you are trying to gain muscle and lose fat, you may want to raise your protein intake from two-thirds of a gram per pound of body weight to as much as 1 gram per pound of body weight. For a 150-pound man, this would mean raising the pure protein intake from 100 to 150 grams, or 15 to 22 ounces of lean chicken, fish, and so on, per day. Remember to consume over three to six meals.

While raising your protein intake will probably lower your testosterone levels, high protein intake can have many benefits for body composition. Protein has been shown to satisfy hunger and speed up the metabolism more than carbohydrates or fats. Protein is also less likely than other calories to be converted and stored as fat. In addition, some studies have shown that higher protein intakes lead to more muscle growth in those who train with weights on a regular basis. The best types of protein for building muscle are those found in milk and eggs.

If your goal is mainly to lose fat, increase your protein intake to 1 gram per pound of body weight and reduce calories from either fat or carbohydrates. I recommend cutting the calories mostly from simple carbohydrates. Try to get all your carbohydrate calories from vegetables, fruits, and high-fiber/unprocessed starches such as whole grains, beans, peas, lentils, and sweet potatoes or yams. Keeping some fat in your diet not only will keep your testosterone levels higher but will help satisfy hunger and keep your energy levels higher while dieting. If you feel a loss of energy while dieting, try the T-booster weight loss program in Chapter 4.

If you are primarily interested in building muscle and are not so concerned about fat loss, you need not cut any calories from carbohydrates or fat when you increase your protein intake. The extra protein will more than likely be used to build new muscle and prevent muscle breakdown while you are on a weight-training program. It is unlikely that any of the extra protein will be stored as fat as long as you are working out regularly. If you are concerned about the small drop in testosterone that may result from higher protein intake, try taking T-boosters before your workouts. (See Chapter 5.)

An added bonus to having a leaner, healthier body is less conversion of testosterone to estrogen. Having excess fat stored on and inside your body also leads to excess estrogen conversion. The most dangerous fat is the kind inside the belly called visceral fat. If your waistline is expanded while the fat rolls are reasonably small, then you have a lot of intra-abominal fat.

While losing weight you may temporarily have a lower testosterone level due to increased aerobic exercise and higher protein intake. But in the long run, a leaner body composition is one of the most healthful ways to balance your testosterone/estrogen ratio.

Exercise

One of the best exercise modes for boosting testosterone levels is brief but intense weight training. If you work out *too* long, your testosterone levels will actually go down. Keep your weight workouts to no longer than twenty to forty-five minutes. Lifting heavy weights with fewer repetitions sends your body a signal to produce more testosterone. So if you are busy and have little time to work out, this is good news. Not only is it unnecessary to work out for less than an hour, but working out longer will actually lower your testosterone levels and may actually impair muscle growth.

You need to plan your program carefully. If you are a beginner at weight training, try starting out with a personal trainer who can suggest appropriate exercises for you. You should engage in weight training three or four times per week. Each workout should emphasize different parts of the body, and you should never work on one part of the body more than once every four or five days. Do two or three sets of no more than ten repetitions to fatigue unless otherwise specified. If you can comfortably do more than ten, increase the weights. Don't wait long between sets. Try to stay a little out of breath to give your body the maximum stimulus for growth.

SAMPLE YIN (HIGH SCORE) WORKOUT PROGRAM

This program should not take you more than forty-five minutes a session.

MONDAY

Bench press, shoulder press, triceps and two other upper body exercises

WEDNESDAY

Leg press, leg extensions, leg curls, calf raises, and two other leg exercises

FRIDAY

Bicep curls, lat pulldowns, sit-ups (four sets, each done in a different way), and two other back-trunk exercises

If you are trying to lose fat, you may be tempted to do a lot of aerobic exercise. While this will accelerate weight loss, it will burn muscle as well. To make things worse, too much aerobic exercise may have negative effects on testosterone levels and testosterone utilization in your body. This can lead to further loss in muscle.

Remember, losing muscle also lowers your body's resting metabolic rate, so it is important to preserve muscle mass while trying to lose fat. Instead of relying on prolonged and intense aerobic exercise, you may consider brisk walking or bike riding. These exercises will burn calories with much less muscle loss and little effect on testosterone levels. You should also engage in regular weight-training that will help burn calories while preserving muscle.

Supplements

Most Americans are deficient in at least one vitamin or mineral. Zinc deficiency can lead to excess conversion of testosterone to estrogen, and proper zinc supplementation can help restore a healthy testosterone-estrogen balance. While taking large doses of zinc will not raise testosterone levels, make sure you get at least 30 milligrams of zinc if you are on a yin sexual mode.

Before taking any T-boosters, you may want to stop taking any T-busters, or sex-busting drugs (see Appendix 2)—substances that inhibit the action of testosterone, decrease its production, or cause it to be more quickly eliminated from the body. For example, we have all been told about the dangers of drinking too much alcohol. However, if more people knew that alcohol could kill their sex lives by increasing the conversion of testosterone to estrogen, would there be less imbibing of alcoholic beverages?

After you have made lifestyle changes to maximize your body's natural testosterone levels, you may still want an occasional boost. High yin types may need extra supplementation. See Chapter 7 for the right Super T Sexual Cocktail for you.

Lifestyle Factors

A stress reaction is a primitive and necessary response for survival, and when you are in a survival stress reaction mode, sex takes the second seat. Stress is perhaps the biggest testosterone buster. Make it a habit to find quiet time to take a break from the stresses of life with family and friends, and make sure you find time for activities that are pleasurable and fulfilling to you. Many people engage in a vicious cycle of stressful living, which lowers their hormone levels, further adding to depression and an edgy mood. Various alternative therapies such as massages and acupressure may also help relieve stress.

Modifications for High Yin Scores

If you are in a high yin sexual mode, the following modifications may be necessary in addition to the core program for proper hormonal balance.

1. Diet: Consume additional MUFAs. Good choices for between-meal snacks are almonds, cashews, macadamia and pistachio nuts, which have a high MUFA content. If you can tolerate it, try taking up to 1/2 tablespoon of virgin olive or almond oil between meals.

2. Exercise more frequently but for shorter durations. Try to make it to the gym for weight training five times a week, but limit your workout to no more than thirty minutes. Don't forget to stretch—it will relax you and boost your testosterone. Since these workouts are short, make them intense, with lower repetitions and higher weights.

SAMPLE WORKOUT PROGRAM FOR MEN AND WOMEN WITH A HIGH YIN SCORE

Each set of four should include one to two low-weight warmup sets of ten to fifteen repetitions, followed by two to three weight-lifting sets with weights that you can lift at maximum three to five times.

MONDAY
    2 to 3 sets of bench presses
    2 to 3 sets of lat pulldowns
    Alternate between the 2 exercises after each set.

TUESDAY
    2 to 3 sets of leg presses or squats
    2 to 3 sets of leg curls
    Alternate between the 2 exercises after each set.

WEDNESDAY
    2 to 3 sets of bicep curls

2 to 3 sets of tricep extensions
Alternate between the 2 exercises after each set.

THURSDAY

2 to 3 sets of abdominal exercises that work the upper, lower, and oblique muscles at the sides. It is important to work the "abs" at least 4 different ways to make sure all the different directions of muscle fibers are stimulated. Keep your spine flat on the floor or straight to reduce back strain. (See Appendix 3, page 237.)

FRIDAY

2 to 3 sets of shoulder presses
2 to 3 sets of calf raises

See the recommendations for T-booster supplementation in Chapter 4 for fat loss, Chapter 5 for muscle gain, and Chapter 7 for enhanced sexuality.

If you have tried these measures and still are suffering from low sexual interest and fatigue and other features that go along with a moderate or high yin sexual mode, you may wish to see a doctor.

Modifications for Women

Two main sources for women's excess estrogen are birth control pills and estrogen replacement therapy. Birth control pills are often silent culprits for women with a low level of sexual interest. Females on a moderate yin sexual mode may wish to consider alternative methods of birth control. Estrogen replacement therapy is often overprescribed and unnecessary for many women who are in good cardiac, brain, and bone health. For women under age sixty, estrogen replacement therapy is probably unnecessary unless there is a strong family history of heart disease, Alzheimer's disease, or osteoporosis. While estrogen therapy may ease hot flashes, these can also be treated with dietary phytoestrogens from sources such as soy products (whole beans, textured vegetable protein, and soy flour are good sources), flax meal, flax flour, lentils, oat bran, triticale, kidney beans, garlic and herbal supplements containing black cohosh, dong quai, soy isoflavones, red clover, and chaste berry.

Yang Lifestyle Strategies: Testosterone-Lowering/Estrogen-Boosting Program

While far more of my patients happen to be on the yin sexual mode, there are some who are in a yang sexual mode. They complain they are preoccupied with sexual thoughts and behaviors, and have sexually driven impulses. They often cannot concentrate on their work and are less productive at their profession than they would like to be. Their mates often become annoyed with their incessant demands for sex, and they, in turn, resort to frequent masturbation. Some on the moderate or high yang sexual mode may be overly aggressive and exhibit hyperactive behaviors.

If you scored a 3 or 4 on the questionnaire in Chapter 7, you are in moderate yang sexual mode and will probably need only the diet and exercise recommendations in the following testosterone-lowering and estrogen-boosting regimen. However, those on the high yang sexual mode (a score of 5 or above) may wish to consider some of the supplements recommended in step 3.

Diet

Eliminate from your diet red meat and saturated fat (found in animal fat and dairy products such as butter, cheese, and baked goods or candy bars with palm or coconut oil). Your testosterone levels probably will fall to more normal levels, and you will have less risk of heart disease and prostate, colon, and other cancers.

Increase the amount of pure protein (protein without fat) in your diet. As mentioned before, high-protein diets lower testosterone levels and are good for building muscle and losing fat. Vegetable sources of protein are especially effective at lowering testosterone and may have many other health benefits as well. Try replacing some of the red meat in your diet with soy products, and supplement with healthy sources of protein (egg whites, vegetable protein, soy protein). Try shakes or smoothies with soy protein, which can lower cholesterol and fight prostate cancer, and has antioxidant effects and can improve your immunity. As added bonuses, soy protein contains phytoestrogens, which can help eliminate some of the negative effects of excess testosterone on your prostate and may even decrease hair loss.

SAMPLE HIGH-PROTEIN, LOW-FAT, LOW-CARBOHYDRATE MEAL PLAN FOR THE YANG (HIGH SCORE) SEXUAL MODE

BREAKFAST

   5 to 10 egg whites scrambled or fried in fat-free cooking spray with lots of spinach and mushrooms. You may add salsa.
   1 to 2 pieces of fruit

LUNCH

   1 to 2 cups of vegetable soup (made with clear broth)
   1 to 2 grilled chicken breast halves
   1 to 2 cups of baked beans with no sugar

DINNER

   Large salad of your choice with fat-free salad dressing
   3 to 6 ounces of grilled fish of your choice
   1 to 2 cups of mixed steamed vegetables
   1 to 2 pieces of fruit

Exercise

Increase cardiovascular exercise and decrease training with heavy weights. Long-duration, exhaustive exercise can lower your testosterone and improve your cardiovascular health at the same time. Regular sessions of prolonged aerobic exercise can also help you relax and may relieve aggressiveness. Good exercises include running, jogging, and cycling. Yoga exercises that emphasize the higher centers of consciousness are helpful. Avoid the ones that concentrate and activate the yoga centers around the sexual organs.

Supplements

The need for extra supplementation may be especially desirable for high yang sexual mode types. Supplements that increase serotonin levels are especially useful. Increasing serotonin has the dual effect of calming you down and lowering your sex drive, ideal for a yang type. One good supplement is 5-hydroxytryptophan (5-HTP), whose effects are similar to the amino acid L-tryptophan (which is available only by prescription). Common doses for 5-HTP are 50 to 100 milligrams one to three times daily on an empty stomach.

Another supplement that may increase serotonin levels is St.-John's-wort. The common dose is 300 milligrams of an extract standardized for .3 percent hypericin (one of the active ingredients in St.-John's-wort) one to three times a day. Do not take other psychoactive substances when on St.-John's-wort. You might also try kava kava, which is most potent as a liquid extract. An effective dose may be 1/2 to 1 teaspoon one to three times a day.

Category 2 T-boosters, or nor-testosterone boosters, may decrease sex drive. Try nor-adione or nor-4-adiol if you want your sex drive to slow down briefly so you can concentrate on other things. The dose ranges are 10 to 50 milligrams for women and 50 to 100 milligrams for men once or twice a day. However, nor-testosterone boosters can also give you more energy, so if you are already somewhat hyperactive, you may want to avoid nor-testosterone boosters. Do not use more than three times a week without medical supervision.

Modifications for High Yang Scores

1. Consume a protein drink in between meals, preferably of a high-quality soy-whey blend.

2. Switch to a primarily vegetarian diet. The food industry has become much better at creating soy- and wheat-based meat substitutes for those who crave meat. Once ridiculed for their taste, soy burgers and soy sausages now can taste remarkably similar to meat and are generally much healthier for a yang type.

3. Exercise aerobically every day for forty-five minutes. This is the best way to calm your nerves and balance your high testosterone levels.

4. Take high-range doses of the supplements recommended. The only caveat is to be careful if you are taking St.-John's-wort and either L-tryptophan and 5-HTP at the same time. If so, you may want to stick to the lower end of the doses.

Modifications for Women

Despite the temptation for a female on a high yang sexual mode to use estrogens, a better alternative might be soy phytoestrogens. These can provide many of the balancing effects of estrogen without the bloating, weight gain, and other side effects of estrogen replacement therapy; in addition, they have a protective effect against breast, ovarian, and other female cancers. Natural progesterone can also help balance the effects of high testosterone levels.

Take It Home

You can balance your body's yin and yang sexual direction in a way that fits your sex and age by simple lifestyle modifications. For those complaining of low sexual interest and lack of energy and drive (yin sexual mode), the program in this chapter is likely to restore testosterone levels. Similarly, those with excessive sexual desire and drive will more than likely enjoy a more balanced and healthy lifestyle with the yang sexual mode program. In either case, you will also reap the rewards of eating a good diet and following a smart exercise program: fewer illnesses, greater mental clarity, and less fatigue, which all lead to better health.

Part IV

Your Personal T-Booster Regimen

- 9 -

Better Body,
Better Sex Day Planner

You are now ready to combine the recommendations outlined in Chapters 4, 5 , 7, and 8 into a personalized Super T regimen that fits your individual profile (gender, age, lifestyle, and goals). This will take only an hour (or less). If you're only interested in T-boosters for sexual enhancement, then your list will be short, and you can essentially confine your review to Chapters 7 and 8. If your goals also include fat loss or muscle gain, you will need to consult Chapters 4 and 5 as well.

Day Planner

Use the following template to create a day-by-day guide to supplements, diet, and exercise. If your primary goal is weight management, focus your energy first on the Fat-Loss Program.

Begin by first calculating your protein, carbohydrate, and fat requirements as outlined in Appendix 1 (page 188), and then create a weekly meal plan. Consult Appendix 3 to build a fat-burning exercise regimen. When you've attained your desired weight, proceed to the Muscle Gain Program.

Consult Chapter 5 for the beginner and intermediate muscle-gain program. You should already be experienced with weight-resistance training before utilizing the supplement regimen recommended in the "Hard-Core" Program.

For the Better Sex T-Booster Regimen, first consult Chapter 7 to determine which T-booster cocktail is right for you. Then create a complete pro-sexual regimen by adding in the recommendations for diet, exercise, and lifestyle that are outlined in Chapter 8.

SUPER T BETTER BODY, BETTER SEX REGIMEN

I. Better Body: Natural Body Makeover

    A. Fat-Loss Program

        1. Calorie-Restricted Days (alternate every 3 days with Maintenance Program)

            Supplements

                T-Boosters _____

                _____

                Miscellaneous Supplements _____

                _____

                Thermogenic Formula _____

                _____

            Exercise

                Aerobic: type/duration _____

                _____

                Anaerobic: type/duration _____

                _____

            Diet

                Total Daily Requirements (in grams)

                    Proteins: _____

                    Carbohydrates:_____

                    Fats: _____

            Meal Plans

                Breakfast

                  Proteins_____

                _____

Carbohydrates _____

_____

Fats _____

_____

Lunch

Proteins _____

_____

Carbohydrates _____

_____

Fats _____

_____

Snack _____

Dinner

Proteins _____

_____

Carbohydrates _____

_____

Fats _____

_____

2. Maintenance Days (alternate every 2 days with Calorie-Restricted Program)

Supplements

T-Boosters _____

_____

Miscellaneous Supplements _____

_____

Thermogenic Formula _____

_____

Exercise

Aerobic: type/duration _____

_____

Anaerobic: type/duration_____

_____

Diet

  Total Daily Requirements (in grams)
   Proteins: _____
   Carbohydrates:_____
   Fats: _____

Meal Plans
  Breakfast

   Proteins_____

   _____

   Carbohydrates _____

   _____

   Fats _____

   _____

  Lunch

   Proteins_____

   _____

   Carbohydrates _____

   _____

   Fats _____

   _____

  Snack _____

  Dinner

   Proteins_____

   _____

   Carbohydrates _____

   _____

   Fats _____

   _____

B. Muscle Gain Program

   1. Beginner to Intermediate

      T-Booster Cycle (alternate with Creatine Cycle every 4 to 6 weeks)

        T-booster supplement _____

        _____

        Exercise _____

        _____

      Creatine Cycle (alternate with T-Booster Cycle every 6 to 8 weeks)

      Creatine Monohydrate

        Loading Phase (first 5 days) _____

        _____

        Maintenance Phase _____

        _____

        Exercise _____

        _____

   2. Hard-Core Program

      On Cycle (alternate with Off Cycle every 6 to 8 weeks)

•➔ *Note:* Lower supplements gradually during the last two weeks. During the last week, begin gradually taking off-cycle supplements.

        T-Booster Supplements for Training Days

        Breakfast _____

        _____

        Lunch _____

        _____

        Workout _____

        _____

        T-Booster Supplements for Non-Training Days

        Breakfast _____

        _____

Lunch _____

_____

Dinner _____

_____

Off Cycle (alternate with On Cycle every 6 to 8 weeks)

Supplement Stack:

Creatine Monohydrate _____

Phosphatidylserine _____

Acetyl-L-Carnitine _____

Optional Supplements:

HMB _____

Ipriflavone _____

Tribulus _____

Others _____

II. BETTER SEX: T-BOOSTER REGIMEN

A. Pro-Sexual Regimen (2 to 5 days prior to lovemaking date)

T-Boosters _____

_____

Other Supplements _____

_____

Exercise _____

_____

Meal Plans

Breakfast

Proteins _____

_____

Carbohydrates _____

_____

Fats _____

_____

Lunch

    Proteins _____

    _____

    Carbohydrates _____

    _____

    Fats_____

    _____

Snack _____

Dinner

    Proteins _____

    _____

    Carbohydrates _____

    _____

    Fats_____

    _____

B. Lovemaking Day Regimen

    T-Boosters _____

    _____

    Viagra (optional)_____

    Other Supplements_____

    _____

    Diet and Exercise Modifications (If any)_____

    _____

~ 10 ~

Medicine Chest

This section is designed to let you be an informed shopper about supplements that improve your sex life and physique.

Many products are combination formulas, containing several T-booster and other ingredients. If you are buying the product to help you build a better body, read Chapter 4 and Chapter 5 and the Muscle Gain and Fat Loss Medicine Chests in this chapter to help you decide what ingredients you need.

If you are buying the product to help you have better sex, read Chapter 7 and the Libido Medicine Chest, and for men, the Sexual Performance Medicine Chest in this chapter to help decide what ingredients you need.

T-Booster Combination Products

Avoid products that combine T-boosters with DHEA or pregnenolone. These two hormones will not make any T-booster program more effective and will likely make it weaker.

Many T-booster combination products have tribulus terrestris and chrysin (5, 7 dihydroxyflavone) in them. Since the effectiveness of these two ingredients has yet to be proven, it is better to take a T-booster by itself before trying a combination product. That way, when you try a combination product you can tell if you get any additional effect from tribulus or chrysin, or if you are better off sticking with a T-booster by itself.

Many T-booster combination products have "protector" ingredients such as saw palmetto in them. Use the Sexual Protector Medicine Chest in this chapter to help you decide which protectors you want in a formula.

Thermogenic Formulas

Almost all thermogenic formulas contain caffeine and ma huang. Look for a product with 100 to 200 milligrams of caffeine per serving. Be especially careful of the amount of ma huang, as this is the most powerful ingredient. A good thermogenic product should have 10 to 20 milligrams of active ephedra alkaloids in the ma huang extract. This can be confusing, as usually you are given an amount of ma huang with a percentage standardized for ephedra alkaloids. To get 10 to 20 milligrams, look for an extract of roughly 150 to 350 milligrams of ma huang standardized to 6 percent ephedra alkaloids.

Many thermogenic products contain other ingredients besides caffeine and ma huang. These include white willow bark, green tea extract, cayenne, and quercetin. Remember that caffeine and ma huang are the strongest ingredients. The other ingredients will only give a marginal increase in effectiveness, so do not pay extra for them.

Some thermogenic products contain synephrine instead of ma huang. This might be a good alternative for people sensitive to ma huang, but remember that synephrine has not yet been proven to be as effective for weight loss.

The rating given to each supplement is based on published human scientific literature as well as clinical experience. Here is what the ratings mean:

A = a supplement considered highly effective within its category and has strong scientific data for the desired effect

B = a supplement that is somewhat effective within its category and has at least some scientific backing for its desired effect

UK = "unknown," a neutral rating because not enough research has been conducted to make a clear-cut judgment

NR = not recommended

Keep in mind that a supplement's grade may vary in different categories. For example, a supplement could score an A rating for muscle building but a B rating for fat loss.

The items that could go into our medicine chest would be endless if one looked at all the touted agents over history. Instead, I have decided to limit items to those that are widely used as well as those with future potential based on logical biochemical premises.

Dose ranges have been provided for all supplements with an A or B rating. These doses are merely general guidelines and are not meant to take the place of your health practitioner's advice. Doses may also be different depending on your age, sex, and medical status. If you are unsure about the correct dose, it is best to start at the low end of the range. This is especially true with all testosterone and nor-testosterone precursors. Always read the warnings on the bottle before using as well. Take the supplements as recommended with food unless otherwise stated.

•← *Caution:* If you have liver or any kidney problems, such as decreased elimination capacity, you need to consult your physician before using supplements in general.

Fat Loss Medicine Chest

Follow these instructions:

- See Chapter 4 for more specific information about how to use these supplements, especially the first four supplements on the list.
- In general, do not use any Category 1 or Category 2 T-boosters more than three times per week.
- If you are on the T-booster fat-loss program in Chapter 4 that requires the use of these supplements four times per week, do not use T-boosters for more than six weeks in a row before taking a six-week break from these supplements.

Supplement	Score for Fat Loss	Dose Range	Expected Effects
Adione (androstene-dione)	B+	Men: 50–200 mg Women: 10–50 mg 1–3 times daily	Same effects as 4-adiol except weaker as an anabolic and androgenic agent. Drawback is that it can be converted directly to estrogen, which can lead to increased fat storage, male breast tissue growth (gynecomastia), or increased estrogen load in both sexes. Anabolic effect: medium Androgenic effect: medium
Caffeine (sources include guarana, kola nut, bissy nut)	B+	100–200 mg, 1–3 times daily	Speeds up metabolism and mobilizes fat. Much stronger when combined with ma huang.

• ➤ *Cautions same as for ma huang.*

Supplement	Score for Fat Loss	Dose Range	Expected Effects
Chitosan (derived from shellfish)	NR		May help prevent fat absorption during food consumption. Attracts fat molecules and binds to them, preventing them from being used by the body for fuel. Probably requires very high doses to have any effect.

• ➤ *Caution:* Prevents normal fat absorption, which reduces absorption of fat-soluble vitamins such as A, D, E, the carotenoids, and possibly alpha lipoic acid and T-boosters.

Supplement	Score for Fat Loss	Dose Range	Expected Effects
Chromium picolinate	B	200 mcg, 1–3 times daily	Moderately effective for weight loss. Good for people with sugar and starch cravings. Can be used for those with glucose metabolism problems.
4-adiol (4-androstenediol)	A	Men: 50–200 mg Women: 10–50 mg 1–2 times daily	Increases strength and energy before workouts and preserves muscle mass while dieting. Women should only take in very small doses. Anabolic effect: high Androgenic effect: High

Supplement	Score for Fat Loss	Dose Range	Expected Effects
Garcinia cambrogia extract (trade names include Citrimax and Citrin)	UK		Fruit extract that may help block the conversion of calories from carbohydrates into fat. May also reduce appetite. No reliable research has been done to prove any of its purported effects.
Guggulsterone	UK		Ancient Indian herb used for weight loss. May increase thyroid hormone levels and thus metabolism. Research done in India has shown this herb to be effective for weight loss, but no Western studies have been done to confirm the effectiveness.
Gynmena silvestre	UK		Indian herb that can help reduce sugar cravings. May lower glucose levels and has been used in the treatment of diabetics.
Ma huang (ephedra)	A	10–20 mg ephedra alkaloids, 1–3 times daily (160–330 mg ma huang standardized to 6% ephedra alkaloids)	May be the most potent fat-loss agent available over the counter: speeds up metabolism, reduces appetite, and increases energy. May cause nervousness in some individuals. Best combined in a standard thermogenic formula with caffeine and white willow bark. Some nasal medications contain ephedrine, one of the strongest active ingredients in ma huang.

• *Caution:* Do not use if stimulant sensitive, anxious, or have heart or blood pressure problems. Always buy from a reputable company and never exceed doses recommended on the bottle.

Nor-adione (nor-androstene-dione)	A–	Men: 50–200 mg Women: 10–50 mg 1–3 times daily	Same effects as nor-4-adiol but not as strong. Anabolic effect: medium Androgenic effect: low

Supplement	Score for Fat Loss	Dose Range	Expected Effects
Nor-4-adiol (nor-4-andro-stenediol)	A	Men: 50–200 mg Women: 10–50 mg 1–3 times daily	Increases energy and preserves muscle mass while dieting. May have fewer side androgenic and estrogenic effects than 4-adiol or adione but won't increase energy as much during weight training. Anabolic effect: high Androgenic effect: low
Norephedrine/ phenylpropanol-amine	A	10–25 mg, 1–3 times daily	One of the active ingredients found in ma huang. Sold both as a supplement (norephedrine) and as an over-the-counter drug (phenylpropalamine) under brand names such as Dexatrim and Accutrim. Less stimulatory than ma huang extract and ephedrine but may be more effective at increasing metabolism and reducing appetite. Avoid time-released formulas; quick-release formulas are more effective and may be safer.

• Cautions same as for ma huang.

Pyruvate (sold both as calcium and sodium pyruvate)	UK		By-product of glucose metabolism in your body. Expensive, and research is inconclusive for its effectiveness.
Soluble fiber supplements (including guar gum, glucommanan, and grapefruit pectin)	A	5 to 15 g before meals	Has been proven effective for weight loss. Helps suppress appetite by creating a feeling of fullness and can stabilize insulin levels. Fiber from a diet high in vegetable and fruits is preferable. Insoluble fiber such as wheat bran also has health benefits but is not as effective for weight loss as soluble fiber. Taking with supple-ments will hinder their absorp-tion.

Supplement	Score for Fat Loss	Dose Range	Expected Effects
Stevia (*Stevia rebaudiana*)	B+	highly variable	Non-toxic. Can be used as a sugar substitute. Can satisfy appetite and sweet cravings without any calories. Extracted from a South American shrub.

Muscle Gain Medicine Chest

Follow these instructions:

- Do not use any Category 1 or 2 T-boosters more than three times per week or more than six consecutive weeks.
- If you are planning on taking higher doses of T-boosters than recommended in this section, be aware of the possible side effects that may occur and consult a physician before beginning such a program.
- If taking higher doses or more frequently than recommended, you should also limit your use of T-boosters to a period no longer than six to eight weeks, followed by an equal period or longer in which no T-boosters are taken.

Supplement	Muscle Building Rating	Dose Range	Expected Effects
Adione (androstenedione)	B+	Men: 50–200 mg Women: 10–50 mg 1–3 times daily	Same uses as 4-adiol except weaker. Drawback is that it can be converted directly to estrogen, which can negate some of the effects of testosterone. Anabolic effect: medium Androgenic effect: medium
ALC (acetyl L-carnitine)	B	500–2,000 mg, 1–2 times daily on an empty stomach	Quasi-amino acid that may help prevent the reduction of testosterone while training. May also improve energy and concentration and have other positive effects on the brain and nerves.

Supplement	Muscle Building Rating	Dose Range	Expected Effects
Chromium picolinate	B	200–600 mcg, in 2 or 3 divided doses	Essential mineral widely sold to use for weight loss. Studies show it can lead to a small increase in muscle mass due to its effect on glucose metabolism.
CLA (conjugated linoleic acid)	B	5–10 g, in divided doses	A fatty acid naturally found in such foods as cheese. Recent human studies have suggested a positive effect on muscle building. May also be an effective antioxidant.
Creatine monohydrate	A	2.5–5 g, 4 times daily for loading 2–5 grams twice daily for maintenance	Amino acid–like substance found in meat that increases strength by increasing the cells' energy production and increases size of muscle cells. Will lead to better workouts and perhaps faster muscle growth. Best taken with a carbohydrate drink. May indirectly be anabolic by increasing cell energy levels and increasing their water content.
DHEA	NR		Abundant, naturally occurring hormone that converts to androstenedione (adione) and 5-adiol in the body. It's better to take adione separately since DHEA combinations can have unpredictable side effects. Although often sold in combination with adione, DHEA can reduce the amount of adione that is converted to testosterone.

Supplement	Muscle Building Rating	Dose Range	Expected Effects
5-adiol (5-andro-stenediol)	UK		May have benefits as an immune system booster. Some research has shown it to be anabolic in laboratory animals. Does not convert to estrogen but has estrogenic effects. Anabolic effect: low Androgenic effect: low
4-adiol (4-androstenediol)	A	Men: 50–200 mg Women: 10–50 mg 1–3 times daily	Great for increasing strength and energy before workouts and promoting muscle growth. Women should only take in very small doses. The strongest of all the pro-hormones. Anabolic effect: high Androgenic effect: high
HMB (beta-hydroxy beta-methylbutryate)	B+	1–3 g, 3 times daily	Amino acid metabolite that might help prevent muscle breakdown during intense exercise. May also help stimulate muscle growth.
Ipriflavone	UK		Similar in structure to phytoestrogens such as soy isoflavones. Used to increase bone mass in Europe and Japan. Results of research that shows it grows muscle in laboratory animals has not yet been proven with human subjects.
Nor-adione (nor-androstene-dione)	A–	Men: 50–200 mg Women: 10–50 mg 1–3 times daily	Same effects as nor-4-adiol but less potent for muscle growth. Anabolic effect: medium Androgenic effect: low
Nor-5-adiol (nor-5-andro-stenediol)	UK		Very little research available. May have estrogenic effects. Anabolic effect: unknown Androgenic effect: unknown

Supplement	Muscle Building Rating	Dose Range	Expected Effects
Nor-4-adiol (nor-4-androstenediol)	A	Men: 50–200 mg Women: 10–50 mg 1–3 times daily	Increases energy and muscle growth. May have fewer side effects than 4-adiol but won't increase strength as much as 4-adiol. Anabolic effect: high Androgenic effect: low
Orchic extract	NR		Extract from animal testicles. May contain small amounts of testosterone, which is poorly absorbed orally. T-boosters are more effective and economical.
Phosphatidyl-serine	B+	100–400 mg, 2 or 3 times daily	Naturally found in soy and in the human brain. May help prevent the increase of the hormone cortisol while training; high cortisol levels can lead to loss of muscle and bone as well as other negative effects.
Pregnenolone	NR		Hormone that is one step removed in the body from cholesterol. Converts into DHEA, progesterone, cortisol and aldosterone. Since it converts into DHEA and, in turn, DHEA converts into androstenedione (adione), it is often sold as part of a combination of testosterone-boosting products. However, since pregnenolone can convert into progesterone, a female hormone, it actually can reduce sex drive and muscle mass.
7-keto DHEA	NR		Hormone very similar in structure to DHEA. Preliminary research indicates it might improve mood and memory, but there is no evidence it has any effect on muscle mass or sex drive.

Supplement	Muscle Building Rating	Dose Range	Expected Effects
Tribulus terrestris	UK		Herbal extract that allegedly boosts testosterone by its effect on the brain. More research needs to be done to be conclusive.

The Libido Medicine Chest

Use these supplements to increase sexual drive and interest and to enhance sexual enjoyment.

•→ *Note:* 4-adiol and adione should not be used more than three times a week.

Supplement	Libido Building Rating	Dose Range	Expected Effects
Adione (androstene-dione)	A−	Men: 50–200 mg Women: 10–50 mg Once a day before sex	Not as strong as 4-adiol for increasing testosterone. May enhance libido and energy by increasing both testosterone and estrogen. Anabolic effect: medium Androgenic effect: medium
Avena sativa	UK		Green oat extract that allegedly increases free-testosterone levels, but no credible medical studies have yet been done.
Beta sitosterol (found in smilax, pygeum, and other herbs)	UK		A plant sterol found in several herbal extracts. Similar action to saw palmetto.
Damiana	UK		Herb touted as "the female Viagra," but there is no good scientific evidence for this effect. May make women less inhibited about sex.

Supplement	Libido Building Rating	Dose Range	Expected Effects
DHEA	B	Men: 5–50 mg Women: 5–25 mg	Naturally occurring hormone that converts into androstenedione (adione) and 5-adiol in the body. Weak libido enhancer for men but a good option for women who are extremely sensitive to androstenedione and 4-adiol.
4-adiol (4-androstenediol)	A	Men: 50–200 mg Women: 10–50 mg Once a day before sex	Perhaps the most potent supplement available over the counter for increasing libido via testosterone boosting. Women should be cautious when taking it—start low and go slow. Anabolic effect: high Androgenic effect: high
Kava kava	B	2–5 ml of a liquid extract, 1–3 times daily	Herbal extract popular in the South Pacific. Sold as a female libido enhancer but affects sexual drive indirectly by relaxing and calming and loosening sexual inhibitions.
L-tyrosine	B	500–1,000 mg, 1–2 times daily, taken on an empty stomach	Amino acid that mildly increases dopamine levels. Most effective when combined with a T-booster. Can increase alertness and energy. Be cautious if you have a skin pigmentation problem or a history of melanoma.
Muara puima	UK		Herb from the Amazonian rain forest. Although there is much anecdotal evidence that this herb boosts libido, more research needs to be done.

Supplement	Libido Building Rating	Dose Range	Expected Effects
NADH (nicotinamide adenine dinucleotide)	B	2.5–5 mg once a day on an empty stomach, 30 minutes to 1 hour before eating	A niacin coenzyme that works as a mild dopamine booster. Best if combined with a T-booster. May need to use daily for at least a week to notice effects.
Nor-adione (19-nor-andro-stenedione)	NR		Will not increase libido. Anabolic effect: medium Androgenic effect: low
Nor-4-adiol (19-nor-4-andro-stenediol)	NR		Will not increase libido. May actually decrease libido if taken in large enough doses. Anabolic effect: high Androgenic effect: low
Oyster extract	NR		Food extract that may help boost testosterone by correcting zinc deficiencies but will not help those who already get enough zinc in their diets. A zinc supplement or a multimineral supplement that includes zinc is a better buy.
Saw palmetto (*Serenoa repens*)	UK		Herbal extract that may indirectly increase sexual pleasure by improving prostate and urinary health. No direct effects on sexuality have been reported.
Tribulus terrestris	UK		Herbal extract that allegedly improves libido by increasing sex hormone levels through its effect on the brain. More research needs to be done.

Supplement	Libido Building Rating	Dose Range	Expected Effects
Yohimbé/ yohimbine	B	5.4 mg yohimbine* or 400–800 mg of a standardized 1% yohimbé extract, 1–2 times daily	Herbal extract from the bark of an African tree that is also the basis of the prescription drug yohimbine hydrochloride. Increases libido through a variety of mechanisms.

•➤ *Caution:* May cause anxiety in some individuals. Avoid if you have problems with high blood pressure. Read all warning labels on the bottle before using. Do not use with Viagra since the combination may cause priapism (prolonged and painful erection lasting for hours that is a medical emergency).

Sexual Performance Medicine Chest

These supplements and drugs are sold for treating male erectile dysfunction. Some of them are being researched on women as vaginal lubrication enhancers as well.

•➤ *Note:* 4-adiol and adione should not be used more than three times a week.

Supplement	Performance Rating	Dose Range	Expected Effects
Ginkgo biloba	B+	40–80 mg, 1–3 times daily	May increase erections by improving blood flow to the penis. Has additional benefits as an antioxidant and a memory booster.
Ginseng (Panax ginseng)	UK		Popular herbal extract that may indirectly improve sexual function through its effects on mood and energy. May also cause anxiety in some people.

* A pharmaceutical drug

Supplement	Performance Rating	Dose Range	Expected Effects
L-arginine	B	2–3 g, 2 times daily	Theoretically may improve blood flow to penis.
Viagra*	A	25–100 mg Once a day before sex	Currently the reigning champion for increasing erections. Expensive but many find it worth the price. May cause headaches and other side effects.

•➤ *Caution:* Exercise extreme caution if heart condition exists and when taking with other medications. Avoid taking with yohimbé or yohimbine.

Supplement	Performance Rating	Dose Range	Expected Effects
Yohimbé/ yohimbine	B+	5.4 mg yohimbine* or 400–800 mg of a standardized 1% yohimbé extract, 1–2 times daily	An herbal extract from the bark of an African tree that is also the basis of the prescription drug yohimbine. Mildly effective. May cause anxiety in some individuals.

•➤ *Caution:* Avoid if you have problems with high blood pressure. Read all warning labels on the bottle before using.

The Sexual Protector Medicine Chest

These supplements may protect you from possible undesirable effects of sex hormones on the hair, skin, prostate, breasts, and other organs.

Supplement	Protection Rating	Dose Range	Expected Effects
Chrysin	UK		A flavone plant compound sold as a supplement to help prevent the conversion of testosterone to estrogen, but has yet to be proven effective.
Fish oil (omega-3 fatty acids)	A	1,000–5,000 mg, 1–3 times daily	Helps lower LDL cholesterol and raise HDL cholesterol and has many other positive effects. An excellent source of essential fatty acids in which most people are deficient.

* A pharmaceutical drug

Supplement	Protection Rating	Dose Range	Expected Effects
Guggulsterone	B	10–30 mg, 3 times daily	Indian herb that may lower cholesterol levels and may also help reduce acne.
High-lignan flaxseed oil	A	1/2–1 tablespoon, 1–3 times daily	Similar effects as fish oil on cholesterol. Lignins from the husks may protect against some of the harmful effects of estrogen.
Indole-3-carbinole	A	400 mg, once daily	Extract from cruciferous vegetables that helps clear the body of harmful estrogen metabolites. Expensive as a supplement but can be found in such vegetables as broccoli, cauliflower, cabbage, and Brussels sprouts.
Pygeum (*Pygeum africanum*)	A–	50–100 mg of a standardized extract, 1–2 times daily	African herb with similar effects as saw palmetto; may improve prostate and urinary problems.
Saw palmetto extract (*Serenoa repens*)	A–	80–160 mg of an extract standardized for fatty acid content, 1–2 times daily	Herbal extract commonly used for prostate and urinary problems. May have an anti-inflammatory effect on the hair and skin.
Soy products (soy protein isolate, soy isoflavones, tofu, tempeh, and others)	A	25–50 mg soy isoflavones daily from any source. Eat at least one serving of a soy food product daily. Whole soybeans are best.	Contain numerous compounds including phytoestrogens, which have a positive regulating effect on the hormonal system and offer protection from prostate and breast cancer. Can reduce LDL ("bad") cholesterol and raise HDL ("good") cholesterol. Soy phytoestrogens do not increase estrogen levels in men, so men need not worry.

Supplement	Protection Rating	Dose Range	Expected Effects
Stinging nettle (*Urtica dioica*)	A–	200–500 mg, 1–2 times daily	Herb with many positive effects on urinary and prostate health. Often found in combination formulas with saw palmetto and pygeum.

·➤ Appendix 1 ➤·

Nutrition

by Cristiana Paul, M.S., Nutrition Director

SPORTS MEDICINE AND ANTI-AGING MEDICAL GROUP

Nutrition Strategies: The Paul System

The strategies presented here can be used to nourish the body to optimal health for a lifetime. Whether your goal is fat loss, muscle gain, maintenance, or sexual enhancement, these guidelines can be adjusted to accommodate any fitness goal and complete a T-booster regimen.

You will not be counting calories for two reasons. One, it is impractical if not impossible for the average person to count calories because most foods (with the exception of those that come prepackaged) are not labeled with the calorie count. Also, the composition of the diet—its protein, carbohydrate, fat, and fiber content—is more important than the caloric values. In other words, the focus should be placed on the quality of the diet, and after that the appropriate portions in each category should be considered.

As a consequence of following the guidelines in this plan, your caloric intake will not go below 70 percent of your basal metabolic rate (BMR) on calorie-restricted (CR) days and will stay around BMR on maintenance (M) days. Keep in mind that theoretical BMR formulas can have an error of plus or minus 30 percent. That is why when following a plan, it is very important to observe the effects of the newly adopted plan and slowly make adjustments until a good rate of fat loss (one to two pounds a week) is achieved.

Now that you understand the basic principle of this eating plan, let's determine the appropriate portions of protein, fat, and carbohydrates for you, based on body weight, percentage of body fat, activity, and goals. Table 1 illustrates the main sources of protein, carbohydrates, and fat. Before you start, it is important that you know your percentage of body fat. If you cannot have it measured by an expert, go to Estimating Your Percentage of Body Fat, page 191, and estimate it from the formula given.

STEP 1: Protein Requirement

Protein should be the first thing you think about when putting together any meal or snack because it

- provides the building blocks for the maintenance and growth of your lean body mass (LBM), which determines approximately 90 percent of your BMR.
- satisfies hunger more than fats or carbohydrates.
- promotes mental well-being by providing precursors for neurotransmitters.
- stimulates much less insulin than carbohydrates and promotes fat oxidation.
- slows down the digestion of carbohydrates, which causes blood glucose levels to rise and fall more slowly, thus stabilizing mood and hunger.

To determine your protein requirement, do the following:

1. Calculate your lean body mass: LBM = (% of body fat) × (Total Weight)
2. Choose an activity factor (AF) of 0.5–1 from Table 5.
3. Determine your daily protein requirement (DP) by this formula:

$$DP = AF \text{ multiplied by } LBM$$

For example, an average female (LBM = 100 pounds) exercising 7 hours per week (AF = 0.75) would require 75 grams (100 × 0.75) of protein per day. An average male (LBM = 200 pounds) who is typically sedentary (AF = 0.50) would require 100 grams (200 × 0.5) of protein per day.

Try to distribute this amount evenly throughout the day. For example:

	Average Female (grams)	Average Male (grams)
Breakfast	20	30
Lunch	20	30
Snack	15	15
Dinner	20	30

Refer to Table 6 for examples of breakfasts, lunches, and dinners based on protein portions of 20, 30, and 40 grams. You will also find suggestions for snacks based on a protein amount of 15 grams. Of course you can put together a snack of 30 grams of protein by doubling everything in that list if that is required to meet your protein requirement. Estimate the required portions of lean protein from Table 2.

STEP 2: Fat Allowance

It is important to have the right amount of healthy fat in every meal or snack because it

- satisfies hunger more than carbohydrates.
- slows down the digestion of protein and carbohydrates, so you feel fuller longer.
- slows down the absorption of carbohydrates and protein, which causes blood glucose levels to rise and fall more slowly, thus stabilizing mood and hunger.
- does not stimulate an insulin response, which is favorable to fat oxidation.

The essential fats (omega-3 and omega-6; see Table 1) also provide building blocks for every cell membrane, brain matter (the brain is 70 percent fat) and important anti-inflammatory hormones.

Establish your fat allowance per meal and snack. An appropriate amount of fat grams is approximately half of the protein grams recommended. Figure 10 grams of fat per meal for the average female and 20 grams of fat for the average male from the examples above and 7 grams for the snacks for both. Refer to Table 4 for examples of typical portions of fat, and Table 1, item 4, for the sources of fat.

Estimate the amount of fat that is in your protein source (fish fat, beef fat, egg yolk, or low-fat vs. skim cheese). Then decide if you can add some fat (low-fat dressing, almonds, etc.) to keep the meal in the moderate-fat zone.

For those pursuing the Super T Fat Loss Program, the recommended amount of protein and fat will be the stable portion of your nutrition plan on maintenance (M) days as well as on calorie-restricted (CR) days. The carbohydrate amount will be the variable portion of your plan, with the higher end on M days and the lower end on CR days.

STEP 3: Variable Carbohydrates

Your optimum amount of carbohydrate is one that will enable fat loss while maintaining the right levels of energy for workouts, muscle gain, and mental focus. All the types of carbohydrate sources are listed in Table 1, item 3. For typical portions of carbohydrates, see Table 3.

Eat as many low-carbohydrate vegetables as you want with a minimum of 6/8 (female/male) servings a day (see Table 1, item 2). These foods have a high content of water, fiber, and phytonutrients and, best of all, are virtually calorie free. You would have to eat thirty cups of spinach or five cups of broccoli to reach the equivalent of one slice of bread. You will have a feeling of satiety, and the absorption of the starches or sugars eaten at the same meal will be slowed down.

Now you are ready to add the other carbohydrates to complete your meal or snack. Choose healthful carbohydrates with unrefined, high-fiber, high-water, and micronutrient content. This includes fruits, legumes (beans, peas, lentils), carrots, whole corn kernels, whole grain products (oatmeal, brown rice, whole grain breads and cereals), and yams (see the first and second column of Table 3). Avoid refined, concentrated, and highly processed carbohydrates, which includes fruit juice or jams, carrot and beet juice, sugary ketchup, refined grain products (white rice, white bread, tortillas, chips, sugary and low-fiber cereals), yogurts, milk, and candy. Don't eat too many potatoes, which have a very high glycemic index even though they are a natural unrefined food. See Table 3 for portions.

In Chapter 4, starting on page 80, and in Table 3 in this Appendix, you are given a range of carbohydrate amount per meal, for example, one to two servings of carbohydrates at a meal. Use the lower end of the carbohydrate range on CR days (for example, one serving) and the upper end of the carbohydrate range (two servings) on the M days. Regardless of the type of day, CR or M, you should try to have no carbohydrates two hours before a cardiovascular exercise in order to promote maximum fat mobilization. If possible, do cardiovascular exercise on an empty stomach, first thing in the morning. If you can't, then do it 2 to 3 hours after a meal or snack.

Before and after weight-training sessions you should always use the upper end of the carbohydrate range on both CR and M days. This is because you need to have glycogen for the workout, and you also want an anabolic state right after the workout, which is favored by higher carbohydrates through the release of insulin. Even though insulin is a suppressor of fat released into the circulation, this is not a priority after weight training because muscle is being built that will burn plenty of fat later, throughout the whole day.

Your carb requirement is between 150 and 200 percent of your DP (Daily Protein Requirement), depending on your activity level. For example, for an average female it is 100 to 150 grams of carbohydrates per day and for an average male it is 150 to 200 grams per day. This translates into 30 to 45 grams of carbohydrates per meal for women and 60 to 80 grams per meal for men. Refer to Table 3 for typical portions of carbohydrates. Keep in mind that some individuals have to reduce carbohydrates by 15 or 30 grams in order to get results (one serving of carbohydrates is 15 grams).

Table 6 contains suggestions for meals with a recommended range for the carbohydrate requirement. This is a starting point for your plan, our best guess; you should allow for slight adjustments on your own.

If you are not losing any weight on CR days with this regimen, either increase the exercise, which is the preferred method, or lower the carbohydrates gradually until you see the desired effect.

On CR days the protein and the fat are the same as on M days, but you can increase these slightly (by 20 percent) to reduce hunger and improve mood/energy.

On M days, both males and females need to add more carbohydrates (15 to 30 grams per meal), just enough to stabilize the weight and not gain back what they have just lost. It takes a bit of trial and error, and your activity levels will be an important determining factor.

Estimating Your Percentage of Body Fat

For women: Measure the following in inches:

Hips around the widest circumference. This is M1.
Abdomen around the belly button. This is M2.
Height without shoes. This is M3.

Look in Table 7:

> Locate measurement M1 in the HIPS column and get the corresponding Constant A.
> Locate measurement M2 in the ABDOMEN column and get the corresponding Constant B.
> Locate measurement M3 in the HEIGHT column and get the corresponding Constant C.

Now you are ready to calculate your percentage of body fat:

> % Body Fat = Constant A + Constant B − Constant C

For men: Measure the following in inches:

> Wrist, where your wrist bends. This is M1.
> Waist at the belly button. This is M2.

Calculate your "Waist minus wrist": $M3 = M2 - M1$.

> Measure in pounds:

> Your weight. This is M4.

> Look in Table 8 and find the pages that contain your "Waist Minus Wrist" measurement, M3.
> Locate the row that contains your weight, M4.

Now you can find your percentage body fat at the intersection between your Weight row (M4) and your "Waist Minus Wrist" (M3) column.

TABLE 1 *Food Group Guide*

1. Protein Sources

| | Animal Origin | | | | Vegetarian Origin | | |
| | | | | | Soybean Based | | |
Meats	Eggs	Milk Yogurt	Cheeses	Protein Powders	Natural	Isolate	Other
chicken	egg white	(also a significant source of carbs)	cottage	whey	soybeans in pod	protein powder	wheat germ†
turkey	egg yolk		ricotta	egg base	roasted soybeans	textured vegetable protein	spirulina (algae)
seafood	Eggbeaters		mozzarella	milk base	soy butter	soy flour cereal	brewer's yeast
beef			cheddar		tempeh	veg. burgers	nuts (almonds, etc.)
veal			Swiss		soy milk	veg. sausages	seeds (sesame, etc.)
pork			provolone		tofu	veg. hot dogs	legumes (peanuts,‡
					soy flour	soy cheese	beans,† peas,†
							lentils†)

2. Vegetables (very low carbohydrate content)

EXAMPLES: salsa, lettuce, spinach, mushrooms, radishes, asparagus, onions, cucumbers, tomatoes, bell peppers, eggplant, squash, broccoli, cabbage, artichokes, bean sprouts, green beans, snow peas, arugula, etc.

The starchy vegetables (carrots, corn, potatoes, yams) fall under the Significant Carbohydrates group because they have a considerable amount of carbohydrates.

(continued)

TABLE 1 (continued)

3. Significant Carbohydrate Sources

Fruits	Legumes	Vegetarian Proteins	Starchy Vegetables	Grains	Milk Yogurts	Sugars
berries	beans	soy-based products	carrots	oat	(also a source of protein)	powders
oranges	peas	(see list above)	corn	rye		bars
peaches	lentils		hominy	barley		shakes
apples	(high in solu-		white potatoes	(high in		sauces
pineapple	ble fiber)		sweet potatoes	soluble		soft drinks
grapes	(contain small		yams	fiber)		alcoholic
juices/jams	amounts of			wheat		drinks
	incomplete			buckwheat		
	protein)			rice		
				millet		
				quinoa		
				(contains		
				some		
				incom-		
				plete		
				protein)		

4. Fat Sources

Monounsaturated*

Avocado	Oils	Nuts
avocado	canola	almonds
guacamole	olive	peanuts
		macadamia

Polyunsaturated*

Vegetarian Source		Animal Source
Oils/Margarine	Seeds/Nuts	
safflower	sesame seeds	yolk
corn	peanuts/almonds	mayo
soybean	soybeans	fish
sunflower	sunflower seeds	

Essential Fats/Oils: Sources of Omega-3

flaxseed oil	brazil nuts
fish oils (fish or capsules)	walnuts

Saturated*

Animal Source		Vegetarian Source
Foods	Fats	
meats	lard	coconut
yolk	butter	palm oil
cheese		cocoa butter
milk		
yogurt		
cream		

5. Cholesterol Sources (minimize consumption)

Egg Yolk	Dairy Fat	Animal Meats
mayonnaise	milk, cheese, butter, cream	beef, pork, lamb, chicken, turkey, fish, shellfish

Note: There is no cholesterol in any vegetarian foods.

* All oils listed are actually a mixture of the three types of fat, but we are grouping them based on what the predominant fat is in each category.
† Also a significant source of carbohydrates.
‡ Also a significant source of fat.

TABLE 2   PROTEIN Content of Typical Portions of Foods

Amt = typical amount; P = protein; C = carbohydrate; F = fat.
The size of a deck of cards of meat weighs 3 oz; a 1-inch cube of any hard cheese weighs approximately 1 oz.

Animal Origin	Amt	P(g)	F(g)	C(g)
Chicken, turkey—white meat	3 oz	20	5	0
Chicken, turkey—dark meat	3 oz	20	10	0
Beef, pork, veal—extra lean	3 oz	20	10	0
Beef, pork—regular	3 oz	20	15	0
Spareribs	3 oz	20	25	0
Tuna/sardines, can, in water	3 oz	20	2	0
Tuna/sardines, can, in oil	3 oz	20	10	0
Lobster, shrimp, clams	3 oz	20	2	0
Sea bass, snapper, flounder	3 oz	20	4	0
Salmon, trout, catfish, swordfish	3 oz	20	8	0
Egg white (4 g protein/piece)	5	20	0	0
Egg yolk	(250 mg cholesterol, 5 g fat/piece)			
Eggbeaters	1/2 cup	12	0	0
Milk, nonfat	1 cup	9	0	12
Milk, low-fat 1%	1 cup	9	2	12
Milk, low-fat 2%	1 cup	9	4	12
Yogurt, nonfat	1 cup	12	0	17[†]
Yogurt, low-fat 1%	1 cup	12	2	17[†]
Yogurt, low-fat 2%	1 cup	12	5	17[†]
Cottage cheese, nonfat	1 cup	30	0	7[†]
Cottage cheese, low-fat 1%	1 cup	30	2	7[†]
Cottage cheese, low-fat 2%	1 cup	30	4	7[†]
Ricotta cheese, nonfat [††]	1 cup	24	0	12
Ricotta cheese, low-fat [††]	1 cup	24	6	12
Ricotta cheese, part skim [††]	1 cup	24	12	12
Mozzarella, Swiss, cheddar, provolone, string cheese)				
nonfat	1 oz	7	0	0
low-fat	1 oz	7	3	0
part skim	1 oz	7	7	0
Protein powders (egg/milk derived)	1 scoop	*	*	*

TABLE 2   *(continued)*

Vegetarian Origin	Amt	P(g)	F(g)	C(g)
Veg. burgers, hot dogs, sausages,	*	*	*	*
pepperoni, chili, tofu pudding, etc.	*	*	*	*
Textured vegetable protein‡	1/4 cup	12	0	3
Soy milk (Mighty Soy)§	1 cup	7	2	8
Soy milk (Eden Soy Extra)	1 cup	10	4	14
Other soy milks (check the carbs)	*	*	*	*
Soy yogurt (Nancy's)//	1 cup	7	4	33
Various soy cheeses	*	*	*	*
Blend of soy/cow milk cheese, such as "Veggie singles" from Soyco	1 slice	4	2	0
Tofu (lite, regular, soft, firm, extra firm)	1/3 cup (3 oz)	6	2	0
Roasted soy nuts	1/4 cup	15	10	10
Nutlettes cereal (from soy flour)#	1/4 cup	12	0	3
Tempeh (soy and brown rice mixture)	*	*	*	*
Soy butter (like peanut butter)	1 Tbs	3	5	5
Soy protein powder, such as	1 scoop	*	*	*
Spirutein (banana, chocolate)	1 packet	15	0	10
Take Care (vanilla, chocolate)**	1 scoop	10	1	3

* Check package for protein content per serving to determine the appropriate portion; also watch for carbohydrates and fat.

† This is the carbohydrate content if no sugar or fruit is added; otherwise, it can be three times as high.

‡ TVP comes in various forms and can be found in health food stores or ordered from 1-800-BEEF-NOT.

§ "Mighty Soy" comes in vanilla, honey, or plain, with variable content of carbohydrates.

// Nancy's is good, and it also has acidophilus cultures.

Order from 1-800-BEEF-NOT.

** Order from 1-800-445-3350.

†† Very good source of calcium, it has 4 times more calcium than cottage cheese!

TABLE 3 CARBOHYDRATE SERVINGS (equal to 15 g of carbohydrates)

FRUITS

Low Carbohydrate Density		*Moderate Carbohydrate Density*		*High Carbohydrate Density*	
apricots	4	apple	1	banana	1/2
black currants	1 1/2 cups	applesauce, unsweetened	3/4 cup	cantaloupe	1 1/2 cups
cranberries	1 1/3 cups	blackberries†	1 cup	grapes†	1 cup
lemon	3	boysenberries†	1 cup	honeydew	1 cup
lime	2	blueberries†	3/4 cup	mango	1/2 cup
nectarine	1 1/2	cherries	15	papaya†	1/2 cup
guava	1 1/2	grapefruit	1/2	pear	1/2
peach, persimmon	1 1/2	fig, raw or dried†	1 1/2	pomegranate	1/2
plum†	1 1/2	kiwi	1 1/2	watermelon	1 1/2 cups
raspberries†	2 cups	orange†	1	fruit juice	1/2 cup
strawberries†	2 cups	pineapple†	3/4 cup	dried fruit (plum, dates)	2 or 3
tangerine†	1 1/2	fruit jam/preserves	2 Tbs	raisins	2 Tbs

VEGETABLE JUICES AND SAUCES

tomato sauce (with no sugar added)	1 cup	tomato ketchup	4 Tbs	V-8 juice	1 1/2 cups
		tomato juice	1 1/2 cups	carrot juice	1/2 cup

STARCHY VEGETABLES (CARROTS, CORN, HOMINY, POTATOES, YAMS)

Whole Kernel Vegetable		*Split Kernel*		*Refined Kernel, Flours*	
corn, kernels	3/4 cup	corn, grits	1/3 cup	cornmeal	1/3 cup
corn on the cob	1/2 ear	popcorn	5 cups	corn tortilla, taco	1 small
carrots, med., raw	3	puffed corn cake	2	corn chips	15
carrots, boiled	1 cup				
carrots, baby	15	*Turns to sugar slowly:*		*Turns to sugar quickly:*	
hominy, kernels	1 cup	sweet potato/yam	1/2 cup	potato, baked/boiled	1/3 med.

LEGUMES (BEANS, PEAS, LENTILS, PEANUTS, ETC.) AND VEGETARIAN SOURCE MILKS

Whole Legume		Mashed Legume		Typically High in Sugars or Starches	
beans (red, black, white)	3/4 cup	beans, refried	1/3 cup	oat milk*	*
chickpeas, lentils	1/3 cup	hummus	1/3 cup	rice milk*	*
peas	1 cup	peas, split	1/3 cup	soy milk (has protein too!)	*

GRAINS (OAT, WHEAT, RICE, RYE, BARLEY, BUCKWHEAT, SPELT, ETC.)

Whole Grains (high fiber and minimal or no processing)		Whole Grain Flours (Some fiber and some processing: milling/puffing)		Refined (White) Flours (no fiber and high processing: husk/germ removed)	
oatmeal (cooked)	1/2 cup	oat bran muffin, small	1	oat flour muffin, small	1
		oat bran muffin, large	1/2	oat flour muffin, large	1/2
muesli (oat flakes)	*	granola (oat flakes plus sugar)	*	oat flour cereals	*
brown/wild rice	1/3 cup	brown rice flour products	*	white rice, noodles	1/3 cup
		brown rice cake	2	white rice cake	2
wheat bread (flourless, whole grain)	1 slice	whole wheat bread	1 slice	white flour bread	1 slice
		whole wheat bagel	1/4	white flour bagel	1/4
wheat berries	1/2 cup	whole wheat pasta	1/2 cup	white flour pasta	1/2 cup
sprouted wheat	1/2 cup	whole wheat pancake	1	white flour pancake	1
		whole wheat English muffin	1/2	white flour English muffin	1/2
		whole wheat roll/biscuit	1	white flour roll/biscuit	1
barley kernels	1/2 cup	whole wheat tortilla, pita	1	white flour tortilla, pita	1
		whole wheat hamburger bun	1/2	white flour hamburger bun	1/2
rye kernels	1/2 cup	pizza/pie crust (9 in)	1/8	pizza/pie crust (9 in)	1/8
whole rye bread	1 slice	whole rye flour bread	1 slice	white rye flour bread	1 slice
Kashi pilaf‡	1/3 cup	Kashi, puffed‡	1 cup	other Kashi cereals‡	*
kasha (buckwheat)	1/2 cup	whole buckwheat pasta	1/2 cup	buckwheat flour pancake	1

(continued)

TABLE 3   *(continued)*

SUGARS

protein bars	*	table sugar, syrup	1 Tbs
honey, fructose	1 Tbs	alcoholic beverages	*

* Check package for carbohydrate content per serving to determine the portion providing 15 g of carbohydrates.
† Contain(s) more phytonutrients.
‡ Kashi is a seven-grain mixture.

TABLE 4   FATS AND OILS

Portions containing 15 g of fat (15 g = 1 Tbs = 3 tsp of oil, fat, cream, heavy sauce, or dressing)

Monounsaturated Oils and Their Sources (most beneficial to health)

Unprocessed Sources	Amt	Cholesterol (mg)	Processed Sources	Amt	Cholesterol (mg)
avocado (med.)	1/3	-	guacamole*	6 Tbs	-
macadamia nuts	5	-	olive oil‡/canola oil	1 Tbs	-

Polyunsaturated Oils and Their Sources (use in moderation)

Unprocessed Sources	Amt	Cholesterol (mg)	Processed Sources	Amt	Cholesterol (mg)
almonds	1/4 cup	-	almond butter	2 Tbs	-
corn kernels	-	-	corn oil	1 Tbs	-
flaxseeds	1/2 cup	-	flaxseed oil	1 Tbs	-
peanuts	1/4 cup	-	peanut oil/peanut butter	1 Tbs/2 Tbs	-
soy nuts	1/3 cup	-	soybean oil/soy nut butter	1 Tbs/3 Tbs	-
sunflower seeds	2 Tbs	-	sunflower/safflower oil	1 Tbs	-
seafood (check protein list for fat)		100 mg/3 oz	margarine, regular§	1 Tbs	†
egg yolks	3	300 mg/piece	fish oil (omega-3 or EPA, DHA)	1 Tbs	†
			mayonnaise, regular	1 Tbs	†

[continued]

201

TABLE 4 (continued)

Saturated Fats and Their Sources (avoid as much as possible)

coconut flakes	3/4 cup	-	coconut/palm oil	Tbs	-
meats; beef, poultry (check protein list)		100 mg/3 oz	lard (from beef, poultry)	Tbs	70 mg/oz
milk, regular	2 cups	20 mg/cup	butter, regular cream	Tbs	70 mg/oz
milk, low-fat, 2%	3 cups	20 mg/cup	cheese, regular (Brie, cream cheese)	1/2 oz	20 mg/cup
milk, low-fat, 1%	6 cups	20 mg/cup	cheese, skim (mozzarella, cheddar, etc.)	2 oz	20 mg/cup
milk, skim	n/a	20 mg/cup	cheese, low-fat (mozzarella, cheddar, etc.)	41/2 oz	20 mg/cup

Note: One easy rule of thumb is that only animal sources of fats and oils may contain cholesterol, depending on how they are processed.
* Quantity depends on brand or on how it's made in a restaurant.
† Quantity depends on brand used. Some take the cholesterol out, some leave it in.
‡ Choose virgin, cold pressed.
§ Choose brands with no trans-fatty acids.

202

TABLE 5 BREAKFAST IDEAS with lowest protein requirement

PROTEIN (20 g)	FAT (10 g)	CARBOHYDRATES† (15–30 g or 1–2 servings)
Category A. Breakfast combinations that allow for protein to be separated from the carbohydrates (easier to vary the carbs)		
1. Omelettes/scrambled eggs (can add lots of vegetables: salsa, mushrooms, spinach, peppers, onions, garlic, cabbage)		
5 egg whites or 3/4 cup Eggbeaters	First account for the fat in the cheese and	1–2 pieces of fruit
3 egg whites + 1 oz hard cheese	meat, and then add:	1/2–1 cup oatmeal
3 egg whites + 1/3 cup ricotta cheese	1–2 egg yolks	1/2–1 cup Kashi pilaf (mixed grains)
3 egg whites + 1 oz turkey/chicken/lox	1–2 tsp oil	1/3–2/3 cup brown or wild rice
3 egg whites + 3 oz tofu or tempeh*	1/4 avocado	1–2 slices whole grain bread
10 oz tofu or tempeh*		1–2 whole grain waffles/pancakes
		1/2–1 whole grain/high-fiber muffin
2. Eggs boiled/egg salad (add celery, pickles, tomato, red bell pepper)		
5 egg whites with mustard (to taste)	1–2 egg yolks 1–2 tsp oil	1–2 pieces of fruit
	1–2 Tbs mayo, light*	1–2 slices whole grain bread
3. Meats or vegetarian imitations		
low-fat turkey/chicken/salmon	First account for the fat in the proteins	1–2 slices whole grain bread
sausages*	used, and then add up to 1 tsp oil.	1/2–1 cup oatmeal
vegetarian sausage,* bacon,*		1–2 whole grain waffles/pancakes
vegetarian patties, burgers*		
4. Low-fat cold cuts and/or hard cheese		
3 sticks low-fat string cheese	First account for the fat in the proteins	1–2 slices whole grain bread
3 oz low-fat mozzarella/provolone	used, then add 1–2 Tbs low-fat cream	
cheese	cheese.*	
3 oz oven-roasted turkey/lox		

(continued)

TABLE 5   (continued) Breakfast Ideas with lowest protein requirement

PROTEIN (20 g)	FAT (10 g)	CARBOHYDRATES† (5–30 g or 1–2 servings)
5. Cottage/ricotta cheese (may add tomatoes, bell pepper, celery)		
2/3 cup low-fat/nonfat cottage cheese	2 Tbs almonds/flaxseeds 1/4 avocado 1–2 Tbs low-fat cream cheese*	1–2 pieces of fruit 1–3 tsp jam
6. Protein shakes (add fiber powder and ice; when using milk and/or juice, account for the carbs/protein added)		
scoops protein powder* (protein powders: whey, casein, soy, rice, pea, or any combination)	1 Tbs peanut butter 2 tsp canola or flaxseed oil 2 Tbs walnuts/flaxseeds	Account for the carbs in the protein powder, and then add: frozen fruit* 1/2–1 cup raw oats
Category B. Breakfast combinations in which protein is combined with carbohydrates		
7. Yogurt combos		
1 cup yogurt plain/lightly sweetened and 1/3 cup low-fat/nonfat cottage cheese or 2 Tbs soy nuts or Nutlettes (soy cereal)	2 Tbs walnuts/flaxseeds 2 Tbs slivered almonds	Account for the carbs in the yogurt.
8. Milk with cereal and soy nuts or Nutlettes		
1 cup nonfat/lowfat milk (cow's or soy) and 2 Tbs soy nuts or Nutlettes (soy cereal)	2 Tbs slivered almonds 1/4 cup soy nuts	whole grain/high-fiber cereal* 1/2–1 cup non-/low-fat milk (cow's soy) 1/4 cup soy nuts/Nutlettes (soy cereal)

204

9. *Oatmeal with protein mixed in*

1½ scoops protein powder with only a few grams of carbs per serving*
¼ cup textured vegetable protein or Nutlettes

1 Tbs peanut butter
2 Tbs slivered almonds

½–1 cup oatmeal
dried fruit*

10. *High-protein pancakes*

2 egg whites and scoop protein powder*
milk*

1 egg yolk
1 tsp oil

whole grain/high-fiber cereal*
½–1 cup raw oats
Account for the carbs in the milk.

11. *High-protein French toast*

2 egg whites and protein powder*

1 egg yolk
1 tsp oil

1–2 slices whole grain bread
sweetener: fructose,* honey,* NutraSweet

(continued)

205

TABLE 5 (continued) BREAKFAST IDEAS with medium protein requirement

PROTEIN (30 g)	FAT (15 g)	CARBOHYDRATES† (15–45 g or 1–3 servings)
Category A. Breakfast combinations that allow for protein to be separated from the carbohydrates (easier to vary the carbs)		
1. Omelettes/scrambled eggs (can add lots of vegetables; salsa, mushrooms, spinach, peppers, onions, garlic, cabbage)		
7 egg whites or 1¼ cups Eggbeaters	First account for the fat in the cheese	1–3 pieces of fruit
4 egg whites + 2 oz hard cheese	and meat, then add:	¹/2–1¹/2 cups oatmeal
4 egg whites + ¹/2 cup ricotta cheese	1–2 egg yolks	¹/2–1¹/2 cups Kashi pilaf (mixed grains)
4 egg whites + 2 oz turkey/	2–3 tsp oil	¹/3–1 cup brown or wild rice
chicken/lox	¹/3 avocado	1–3 slices whole grain bread
5 egg whites + 4 oz tofu or tempeh*		1–3 whole grain waffles/pancakes
15 oz tofu or tempeh*		¹/2–1 whole grain/high-fiber muffin
2. Eggs boiled/egg salad (add celery, pickles, tomato, red bell pepper)		
7 egg whites with mustard (to taste)	1–2 egg yolks	1–3 pieces of fruit
	1–2 Tbs mayo, light*	1–3 slices whole grain bread
3. Meat or vegetarian imitations		
low-fat turkey/chicken/salmon	First account for the fat in the proteins	1–3 slices whole grain bread
sausages*	used, and then add up to 2 tsp oil.	¹/2–1 cup oatmeal
vegetarian sausage,* bacon,*		1–2 whole grain waffles/pancakes
vegetarian patties, burgers*		

206

4. *Low-fat cold cuts and/or hard cheese*

4 sticks low-fat string cheese
4 oz low-fat mozzarella/provolone cheese
4 oz oven-roasted turkey/lox

First account for the fat in the proteins used, then add 2–3 Tbs low-fat cream cheese.*

1–3 slices whole grain bread

5. *Cottage/ricotta cheese [may add tomatoes, bell pepper, celery]*

1 cup low-fat/nonfat cottage cheese

3 Tbs almonds/flaxseeds
$^1/_3$ avocado
2–3 Tbs low-fat cream cheese*

1–3 pieces of fruit
1–5 tsp jam

6. *Protein shakes (add fiber powder and ice; when using milk and/or juice, account for the carbs/protein added)*

1 scoop protein powder*
(protein powders: whey, casein, soy, rice, pea, or any combination)

2 Tbs peanut butter
3 tsp canola or flaxseed oil
3 Tbs walnuts/flaxseeds

Account for the carbs in the protein powder, and then add:
frozen fruit*
$^1/_2$–$1^1/_2$ cups raw oats

Category B. Breakfast combinations in which protein is combined with carbohydrates

7. *Yogurt combos*

1 cup yogurt, plain or lightly sweetened, and $^1/_2$ cup low-fat/nonfat cottage cheese or $^1/_4$ cup soy nuts or Nutlettes (soy cereal)

3 Tbs walnuts/flaxseeds
$^1/_4$ cup slivered almonds

Account for the carbs in the yogurt.

8. *Milk with cereal and soy nuts or Nutlettes*

1 cup nonfat/low-fat milk (cow's or soy) and $^1/_3$ cup soy nuts or Nutlettes (soy cereal)

$^1/_4$ cup slivered almonds
$^1/_3$ cup soy nuts

whole grain/high-fiber cereal*
$^1/_2$–$1^1/_2$ cups non-/low-fat milk (cow's/soy)
$^1/_3$ cup soy nuts/Nutlettes (soy cereal)

(continued)

TABLE 5 *(continued)*   Breakfast Ideas with medium protein requirement

PROTEIN (30 g)	FAT (15 g)	CARBOHYDRATES† (15–45 g or 1–3 servings)
9. Oatmeal with protein mixed in		
2 scoops protein powder with only a few grams of carbs per serving* ¹/2 cup textured vegetable protein or Nutlettes	2 Tbs peanut butter ¹/4 cup slivered almonds	¹/2–1¹/2 cups oatmeal dried fruit*
10. High–protein pancakes		
3 egg whites and scoop protein powder* milk*	1–2 egg yolks 1–2 tsp oil	whole grain/high-fiber cereal* ¹/2–1¹/2 cups raw oats Account for the carbs in the milk.
11. High–protein French toast		
3 egg whites and protein powder*	1–2 egg yolks 1–2 tsp oil	1–3 slices whole grain bread sweetener: fructose* honey,* NutraSweet

TABLE 5 (continued) BREAKFAST IDEAS with highest protein requirement

PROTEIN (40 g)	FAT (20 g)	CARBOHYDRATES† (30–60 g or 2–4 servings)
Category A. Breakfast combinations that allow for protein to be separated from the carbohydrates (easier to vary the carbs)		
1. Omelettes/scrambled eggs (can add lots of vegetables: salsa, mushrooms, spinach, peppers, onions, garlic, cabbage)		
10 egg whites or 1³/4 cups Eggbeaters 6 egg whites + 2 oz hard cheese 6 egg whites + 1/2 cup ricotta cheese 6 egg whites + 2 oz turkey/chicken/lox 7 egg whites + 6 oz tofu or tempeh* 20 oz tofu or tempeh*	First account for the fat in the cheese and meat, then add: 1–2 egg yolks 2–3 tsp oil 1/2 avocado	2–4 pieces of fruit 1–2 cups oatmeal 1–2 cups Kashi pilaf (mixed grains) 2/3–1¹/3 cups brown or wild rice 2–4 slices whole grain bread 2–4 whole grain waffles/pancakes 1 whole grain/high-fiber muffin
2. Eggs boiled/egg salad (add celery, pickles, tomato, red bell pepper)		
10 egg whites with mustard (to taste)	2 egg yolks 2 Tbs mayo, light	2–4 pieces of fruit 2–4 slices whole grain bread
3. Meats or vegetarian imitations		
low-fat turkey/chicken/salmon sausages* vegetarian sausage,* bacon,* vegetarian patties, burgers*	First account for the fat in the proteins used, then add up to 1 Tbs oil.	2–4 slices whole grain bread 1/2–1 cup oatmeal 1–2 whole grain waffles/pancakes
4. Low-fat cold cuts and/or hard cheese		
6 sticks low-fat string cheese 6 oz low-fat mozzarella/provolone cheese 6 oz oven-roasted turkey/lox	First account for the fat in the proteins used, then add 3–4 Tbs low-fat cream cheese.*	2–4 slices whole grain bread
		(continued)

TABLE 5 (continued) Breakfast Ideas with highest protein requirement

PROTEIN (40 g)	FAT (20 g)	CARBOHYDRATES† (30–60 g or 2–4 servings)
5. Cottage/ricotta cheese (may add tomatoes, bell pepper, celery)		
1¹/3 cups low-fat/nonfat cottage cheese	4 Tbs almonds/flaxseeds ¹/3 avocado 3–4 Tbs low-fat cream cheese*	2–4 pieces of fruit 1–2 Tbs jam
6. Protein shakes (add fiber powder and ice; when using milk and/or juice, account for the carbs/protein added)		
scoops protein powder* (protein powders: whey, casein, soy, rice, pea, or any combination)	3 Tbs peanut butter 4 tsp canola or flaxseed oil 4 Tbs walnuts/flaxseeds	Account for the carbs in the protein pow- der, and then add frozen fruit* 1–2 cups raw oats
Category B. Breakfast combinations in which protein is combined with carbohydrates		
7. Yogurt combos		
1 cup yogurt, plain or lightly sweetened, and 1 cup low-fat/nonfat cottage cheese or ¹/4 cup soy nuts or Nutlettes (soy cereal)	4 Tbs walnuts/flaxseeds ¹/3 cup slivered almonds	Account for the carbs in the yogurt.
8. Milk with cereal and soy nuts or Nutlettes		
1¹/2 cups nonfat/low-fat milk (cow's or soy) and ¹/3 cup soy nuts or Nutlettes (soy cereal)	¹/3 cup slivered almonds ¹/3 cup soy nuts	whole grain/high-fiber cereal* 2 cups nonfat/low-fat milk (cow's/soy) ¹/3 cup soy nuts/Nutlettes (soy cereal)

9. *Oatmeal with protein mixed in*

2½ scoops protein powder with only a few grams of carbs per serving*
½ cup textured vegetable protein or Nutlettes
3 Tbs peanut butter
⅓ cup slivered almonds
1–2 cups oatmeal
dried fruit*

10. *High-protein pancakes*

5 egg whites and scoop protein powder*
milk*
2 egg yolks
2 tsp oil
whole grain/high-fiber cereal*
1–2 cups raw oats
Account for the carbs in the milk.

11. *High-protein French toast*

5 egg whites and protein powder*
2 egg yolks
2 tsp oil
2–4 slices whole grain bread
sweetener: fructose,* honey,* NutraSweet

* Figure out the quantity you need based on product labels, to meet the required amount of protein, fat, or carbohydrates.
† If you want to eliminate carbohydrates at breakfast to speed up fat burning, use a fiber cracker with a few grams of carbohydrates, such as Bran-a-Crisp, Wasa, or Ak-Mak.

(continued)

TABLE 5 (continued) LUNCH OR DINNER IDEAS with lowest protein requirement

PROTEIN (20 g)	FAT (15 g)	CARBOHYDRATES (15–30 g or 1–2 servings of 15 g)
1. Salad (with lots of greens and a protein source)		
3 oz chicken/turkey/lox/tuna	Account for the fat in the meat, cheese,	1–2 pieces of fruit
3 oz shrimp/lobster/crab meat/	egg, tofu, tempeh, soybeans, then add:	1–2 cups carrots
sardines	2 tsp regular dressing	1/2–1 1/2 cups corn
3 oz low-fat/nonfat hard cheese	2 Tbs low-fat dressing*	1–2 cups peas
3 oz low-fat/nonfat soy cheese	1/4 cup walnuts/almonds	3/4–1 1/2 cups regular beans†
5 boiled egg whites (egg salad)	1/3 avocado	1/2–1 cup Kashi pilaf/puffed
tofu/tempeh*	1–2 egg yolks	1/3–2/3 cup brown or wild rice
1/4 cup soy nuts (roasted soybeans)		1–2 slices whole grain bread
1 cup black soybeans		a few high-fiber crackers*
1 1/2 cups green soybeans		
2. Baked/poached/grilled protein with sides of vegetables, starches (add green salad or vegetable soup to make the meal more filling and nutritious)		
3 oz chicken/turkey/lox/tuna	2 tsp regular dressing/sauce	Same options as in example 1 and occa-
3 oz shrimp/lobster	low-fat dressing sauce*	sionally but not preferably:
tofu/tempeh*		1/3–2/3 baked potato
		1/2–1 cup mashed potatoes
3. Chinese stir-fry (with lots of vegetables; go light on the oil or sweet sauces)		
3 oz chicken/lean beef, shrimp	2 tsp oil	1/3–2/3 cup brown or wild rice
tofu/tempeh*		1 rice flour wrap
1/4 cup soy nuts (roasted soybeans)		Same options as in example 1

212

4. *Vegetable soup/chilli [lots of light vegetables: tomatoes, onions, green beans, cabbage, zucchini]*

3 oz chicken/turkey/lean beef tofu/tempeh*	2 tsp oil	Same options as in example 1
1/2 cup textured vegetable protein 1 cup black soybeans 1 1/2 cups green soybeans		3/4–1 1/2 cups regular beans‡ 1/3–2/3 cup lentils

5. *Japanese soba/udon [lots of vegetables: bean sprouts, cabbage, etc.)*

3 oz chicken/shrimp tofu*	2 tsp oil	1/2–1 cup noodles Same options as in example 1

6. *Mexican food (use lots of salsa and lettuce, cabbage for appetizer, preferably marinated carrot sticks)*

Fajitas/Tacos/Burrito/Tostada 3 oz chicken/turkey/lean beef/fish Albondigas soup (meatballs and vegetables)	2 tsp oil 1/3 avocado or some guacamole* 1 oz regular cheese 2–3 oz non-fat/low-fat cheese avoid sour cream	1–2 cups marinated carrots 3/4–1 1/2 cups regular beans‡ 1/3–2/3 cup regular beans, refried‡ 15–20 chips (preferably baked) 1–2 tortillas/1–2 tacos/1/2–1 tostada 1/3–2/3 cup rice, pref. brown or wild Same options as in example 1

7. *Italian food [start with minestrone soup, roasted bell peppers, not white bread]*

Eggplant Parmigiana/Lasagna† 1 cup low-fat/nonfat ricotta 3 oz low-fat/nonfat mozzarella tofu* Pasta† 3 oz chicken/lean beef/shrimp/salmon tofu/tempeh* 1 1/2 cups textured vegetable protein	Account for the fat in the cheese, and then add some oil.	Same options as in example 1 1–2 slices bread pasta*

(continued)

213

TABLE 5 *(continued)* Lunch or Dinner Ideas with lowest protein requirement

PROTEIN (20 g)	FAT (15 g)	CARBOHYDRATES (15–30 g or 1–2 servings of 15 g)
8. Sandwich (with lots of vegetables, and add green salad or vegetable soup to make the meal more filling and nutritious)		
3 oz chicken/turkey/lox/tuna tofu/tempeh*	1–2 Tbs light cream cheese*	Same options as in example 1
vegetarian burgers* (high protein)	2 tsp regular cream cheese	fiber crackers*
3 oz low-fat/nonfat hard cheese	1–2 Tbs light mayonnaise*	1–2 slices whole grain bread
3 oz low-fat/nonfat soy cheese	2 tsp regular mayonnaise	
	2 tsp oil	

TABLE 5 (continued)   LUNCH OR DINNER IDEAS with medium protein requirement

PROTEIN (30 g)	FAT (15 g)	CARBOHYDRATES (15–45 g or 1–3 servings of 15 g)
1. Salad (with lots of greens and a protein source)		
4 oz chicken/turkey/lox/tuna	Account for the fat in the meat, cheese,	1–3 pieces of fruit
4 oz shrimp/lobster/crab meats/sardines	egg, tofu, tempeh, soybeans, then add:	1–3 cups carrots
7 boiled egg whites (egg salad)	1 Tbs regular dressing	³/4–2 cups corn
4 oz low-fat/nonfat hard cheese	2–3 Tbs ow-fat dressing*	1–3 cups peas
4 oz low-fat/nonfat soy cheese	¹/4 cup walnuts/almonds	³/4–2 cups regular beans‡
tofu/tempeh*	¹/3 avocado	¹/2–1¹/2 cups Kashi pilaf/puffed
¹/4 cup soy nuts (roasted soybeans)	1–2 egg yolks	¹/3–1 cup brown or wild rice
1¹/2 cups black soybeans		1–3 slices bread
green soybeans*		a few high-fiber crackers*
2. Baked/poached/grilled protein with sides of vegetables, starches (add green salad or vegetable soup to make the meal more filling and nutritious)		
4 oz chicken/turkey/lox tuna	1 Tbs regular dressing/sauce	Same options as in example 1 and
4 oz shrimp/lobster	2–3 Tbs low fat dressing*	occasionally but not preferably:
tofu/tempeh*		¹/3–1 baked potato
		¹/2–1¹/2 cups mashed potatoes
3. Chinese stir-fry (with lots of vegetables; go light on the oil or sweet sauces)		
4 oz chicken/lean beef or shrimp	1 Tbs oil	¹/3–1 cup brown or wild rice
tofu/tempeh*		1–3 rice flour wraps
¹/3 cup soy nuts (roasted soybeans)		Same options as in example 1

(continued)

215

TABLE 5 (continued)   Lunch or Dinner Ideas with medium protein requirement

PROTEIN (30 g)	FAT (15 g)	CARBOHYDRATES (15–45 g or 1–3 servings of 15 g)
4. Vegetable soup/chili [lots of light vegetables: tomatoes, onions, green beans, cabbage, zucchini]		
4 oz chicken/turkey/lean beef tofu/tempeh* 2¹/2 cups textured vegetable protein 1¹/2 cups black soybeans 2¹/2 cups green soybeans	1 Tbs oil	Same options as in example 1 3/4–2 cups regular beans‡ ¹/3–1 cup lentils
5. Japanese soba/udon [lots of vegetables: bean sprouts, cabbage, etc.)		
4 oz chicken/shrimp tofu*	1 Tbs oil	Same options as in example 1 ¹/2–1¹/2 cups noodles
6. Mexican food (use lots of salsa, lettuce, and cabbage; for appetizer, preferably marinated carrot sticks)		
Fajitas/Tacos/Burrito/Tostada 4 oz chicken/turkey/lean beef/fish Albondigas soup (meatballs and vegetables)	1 Tbs oil ¹/3 avocado or some guacamole* 1¹/2 oz regular cheese 3–4 oz skim/low-fat cheese avoid sour cream	Same options as in example 1 1–3 cups marinated carrots 15–45 chips (hopefully baked) 1–3 tortillas/ 1–3 tacos/ ¹/2 tostadas ¹/3–1 cup rice, pref. brown or wild 3/4–2 cups regular beans‡ ¹/3–1 cup regular beans, refried‡

216

7. Italian food [start with minestrone soup, roasted bell peppers, not white bread]

Eggplant Parmigiana/lasagna†	Account for the fat in the cheese, and	Same options as in example 1
1.3 cups low-fat/nonfat ricotta	then add some oil.	1–3 slices bread
4 oz low-fat/nonfat mozzarella		pasta*
tofu*		
Pasta†		
4 oz chicken/lean beef/shrimp/salmon		
tofu/tempeh*		
2¹/2 cups textured vegetable protein		

8. Sandwich [with lots of vegetables, and add green salad or vegetable soup to make the meal more filling and nutritious]

4 oz chicken/turkey/lox tuna	2–3 Tbs light cream cheese*	Same options as in example 1
tofu/tempeh*	1 Tbs regular cream cheese	fiber crackers*
vegetarian burgers* (high protein)	1–2 Tbs light mayonnaise*	1–3 slices whole grain bread
4 oz low-fat/nonfat hard cheese	1 Tbs regular mayonnaise	
4 oz low-fat nonfat soy cheese	1 Tbs oil	

(continued)

TABLE 5 (continued) LUNCH OR DINNER IDEAS with highest protein requirement

PROTEIN (40 g)	FAT (20 g)	CARBOHYDRATES [30–60 g or 2–4 servings of 15 g]
1. Salad (with lots of greens and a protein source)		
6 oz chicken/turkey/lox/tuna	Account for the fat in the meat, cheese,	2–4 pieces of fruit
6 oz shrimp/lobster/crab meat/	egg, tofu, tempeh, soybeans, then add:	2–4 cups carrots
sardines	1½ Tbs regular dressing	1½–3 cups corn
10 boiled egg whites (egg salad)	¾ Tbs low-fat dressing*	2–4 cups peas
6 oz low-fat/nonfat hard cheese	⅓ cup walnuts/almonds	1½–2 cups regular beans‡
6 oz low-fat/nonfat soy cheese	⅓ avocado	1–2 cups Kashi pilaf/puffed
tofu/tempeh*	1–2 egg yolks	⅔–1½ cups brown or wild rice
⅓ cup soy nuts (roasted soybeans)		2–4 slices bread
2 cups black soybeans		a few high-fiber crackers*
3½ cups green soybeans		
2. Baked/poached/grilled protein with sides of vegetables, starches (add green salad or vegetable soup to make the meal more filling and nutritious)		
6 oz chicken/turkey/lox/tuna	1½ Tbs regular dressing/sauce	Same options as in example 1 and occa-
6 oz shrimp/lobster	3–4 Tbs low-fat dressing*	sionally but not preferably:
tofu/tempeh*		⅔–1⅓ baked potatoes
		1–2 cups mashed potatoes
3. Chinese stir-fry (go light on the oil or sweet sauces)		
6 oz chicken/lean beef/shrimp	1½ Tbs oil	⅔–1½ cups brown or wild rice
tofu/tempeh*		2–4 rice flour wraps
⅔ cup soy nuts (roasted soybeans)		Same options as in example 1

218

4. *Vegetable soup/chili [lots of light vegetables: tomatoes, onions, green beans, cabbage, zucchini]*

6 oz chicken/turkey/lean beef tofu/tempeh*	1¹/2 Tbs oil	Same options as in example 1
3 cups textured vegetable protein		1¹/2–3 cups regular beans‡
2 cups black soybeans		2/3–1¹/3 cups lentils
3¹/2 cups green soybeans		

5. *Japanese soba/udon [lots of vegetables: bean sprouts, cabbage, etc.]*

6 oz chicken/shrimp tofu*	1¹/2 Tbs oil	Same options as in example 1
		1–2 cups noodles

6. *Mexican food [use lots of salsa and lettuce, cabbage for appetizer, preferably marinated carrot sticks]*

Fajitas/Tacos/Burrito/Tostada	1¹/2 Tbs oil	Same options as in example 1
6 oz chicken/turkey/lean beef/fish	1/3 avocado or some guacamole*	2–4 cups marinated carrots
Albondigas soup (meatballs and vegetables)	2 oz regular cheese	30–60 chips (preferably baked)
	4–5 oz low-fat/nonfat cheese*	2–4 tortillas/2–4 tacos/1–2 tostadas
	avoid sour cream	2/3–1¹/3 cups rice, pref. brown or wild
		1¹/2–3 cups regular beans‡
		2/3–1¹/3 cups regular beans, refried‡

(continued)

219

TABLE 5 (continued) Lunch or Dinner Ideas with highest protein requirement

PROTEIN (40 g)	FAT (20 g)	CARBOHYDRATES (30–60 g or 2–4 servings of 15 g)
7. Italian food (start with minestrone soup, roasted bell peppers, not white bread)		
Eggplant Parmigiana/Lasagna†	Account for the fat in the cheese, and then add some oil.	Same options as in example 1
1²/3 cups low-fat/nonfat ricotta		2–4 slices bread
6 oz low-fat/nonfat mozzarella		pasta*
tofu*		
Pasta†		
6 oz chicken/lean beef/shrimp/salmon		
tofu/tempeh*		
2¹/2 cups textured vegetable protein		
8. Sandwich (with lots of vegetables, and add green salad or vegetable soup to make the meal more filling and nutritious)		
6 oz chicken/turkey/lox tuna	3–4 Tbs light cream cheese*	Same options as in example 1
tofu/tempeh*	1¹/2 Tbs regular cream cheese	fiber crackers*
vegetarian burgers* (high protein)	3–4 Tbs light mayonnaise*	2–4 slices whole grain bread
6 oz low-fat/nonfat hard cheese	1¹/2 Tbs regular mayonnaise	
6 oz low-fat/nonfat soy cheese	1¹/2 Tbs oil	

* Figure out the quantity you need based on product labels, to meet the required amount of protein, fat, or carbohydrates.
† Choose pasta made from whole grains, enriched with protein and vegetables; quantity depends on the brand used.
‡ "Regular beans" include kidney, black, and white beans. Do not include green beans, which fall under low-carbohydrate vegetables, or soybeans.

TABLE 5 (continued) SNACK IDEAS with medium protein requirement

PROTEIN (15 g)	FAT (5 g)	CARBOHYDRATES (15 g)
1. Cheese snacks		
1/2 cup cottage cheese[†]	Account for the fat in the cheese.	1 piece of fruit
1/2 cup ricotta cheese	May add 2 Tbs walnuts/slivered almonds.	1 slice of whole grain bread
2 sticks low-fat string cheese		a few high-fiber crackers[*]
2 oz nonfat/low-fat cheese (cheddar, provolone, mozzarella, soy)		1/2 whole grain, low-fat, high-fiber muffin
2. Meat or vegetarian meat (add a bell pepper or tomato)		
2 oz oven-roasted turkey	2 Tbs low-fat cream cheese	1 slice whole grain bread
2 oz lox		a few high-fiber crackers[*]
vegetarian imitations		
3. Turkey/beef/tuna/salmon jerky or sardines		
Check package for amount of protein.		Same as above
4. Sardines or herring		
Check package for amount of protein.	Drain the oil if any.	Same as above
5. Yogurt combos		
1/2–1 cup low-fat/nonfat yogurt, plain or lightly sweetened, and 1/2 cup low-fat/nonfat cottage cheese or 1/8–1/4 cup soy nuts or Nutlettes (soy cereal)	Account for the fat included with the cheese, yogurt, or soy nuts. May add 2 Tbs walnuts/slivered almonds.	The yogurt may contain a lot of carbohydrates, depending on the brand.

(continued)

TABLE 5 (continued) Snack Ideas with medium protein requirement

PROTEIN (15 g)	FAT (5 g)	CARBOHYDRATES (15 g)
6. Soy nuts or green soybeans in the pod		
1/2 cup green soybeans 1/4 cup soy nuts	The soybeans have between 5 and 10 g of fat per serving.	1 piece of fruit 1 cup applesauce
7. Protein shakes *(add fiber powder to make them more filling)*		
When using milk, account for the protein added. scoop protein powder* (protein powders: whey, casein, soy, rice, pea, or any combination)	Account for the fat in the milk or yogurt, if any, and then add: 1 Tbs peanut/soy nut butter 2 Tbs walnuts/slivered almonds 1 Tbs canola oil 2 tsp flaxseed oil	When using milk, juice, yogurt, account for the carbs added (milk has 12 g carbs/cup; yogurt has 16–45 g carbs/cup; juice has 25–40 g carbs/cup). Account for the carbs in the protein powder if significant. May add 1 piece of fresh fruit, 1 cup frozen fruit or applesauce, 1/2 cup raw oats.
8. Protein bars		
a. High-protein/moderate carbohydrate bars (per bar: 15 g protein, 20 g carbs, 5 g fat) b. High-protein/low-carbohydrate bars (per bar: 30 g protein, 9–15 g carbs, 5 g fat) Have 1/2 bar.		

* Figure out the quantity you need based on product labels, to meet the required amount of protein, fat, or carbohydrate.
† If fruit and sweeteners added, account for the carbohydrates.

TABLE 6   Activity Factor Criteria for Protein Requirement

1. *AF = 0.5* for the typical *sedentary* individual who does not engage in any regular physical activity and whose job requires mostly sitting.
2. *AF = 0.6* for the *moderately active* individual who is exercising *moderately* for thirty minutes three times per week, or the person's job requires walking thirty minutes per day.
3. *AF = 0.7* for the *active* individual who is exercising *moderately* for thirty minutes six times a week, or the person's job requires walking one hour a day or lifting heavy objects thirty minutes per day. (This could include a homemaker who does household chores and/or lifts small children.)
4. *AF = 0.8* for the *very active* individual who is exercising *moderately* for one hour or *intensively* for thirty minutes, six or seven times per week, or the person's job requires walking two hours a day or lifting one hour a day.
5. *AF = 0.9* for the *typical athlete* who is exercising *moderately* for two hours or *intensively* for one hour, six or seven times per week, or the person's job requires walking four hours a day or lifting two hours a day.
6. *AF = 1 or more* for the *elite athlete* who is engaged in competitive endurance or strength training or is a very physical worker engaged in mining, construction, and so forth.

Moderate physical exertion corresponds to a heart rate of 55 to 70 percent of your maximum heart rate or light weight lifting (15 to 20 repetitions per set).
Intense physical exertion corresponds to a heart rate of 70 to 85 percent of your maximum heart rate or heavy weight lifting (6 to 8 repetitions per set).
Note: Your maximum heart rate equals 220 minus your age.

TABLE 7 BODY FAT CALCULATION—WOMEN

Conversion Constants to Predict Percentage of Body Fat—Women

HIPS		ABDOMEN		HEIGHT	
(M1) Inches	Constant A	(M2) Inches	Constant B	(M3) Inches	Constant C
30	33.48	20	14.22	55	33.52
30.5	33.83	20.5	14.40	55.5	33.67
31	34.87	21	14.93	56	34.13
31.5	35.22	21.5	15.11	56.5	34.28
32	36.27	22	15.64	57	34.74
32.5	36.62	22.5	15.82	57.5	34.89
33	37.67	23	16.35	58	35.35
33.5	38.02	23.5	16.53	58.5	35.50
34	39.06	24	17.06	59	35.96
34.5	39.41	24.5	17.24	59.5	36.11
35	40.46	25	17.78	60	36.57
35.5	40.81	25.5	17.96	60.5	36.72
36	41.86	26	18.49	61	37.18
36.5	42.21	26.5	18.67	61.5	37.33
37	43.25	27	19.20	62	37.79
37.5	43.60	27.5	19.38	62.5	37.94
38	44.65	28	19.91	63	38.40
38.5	45.00	28.5	20.09	63.5	38.55
39	46.05	29	20.62	64	39.01
39.5	46.40	29.5	20.80	64.5	39.16
40	47.44	30	21.33	65	39.62
40.5	47.79	30.5	21.51	65.5	39.77
41	48.84	31	22.04	66	40.23
41.5	49.19	31.5	22.22	66.5	40.38
42	50.24	32	22.75	67	40.84
42.5	50.59	32.5	22.93	67.5	40.99
43	51.64	33	23.46	68	41.45
43.5	51.99	33.5	23.64	68.5	41.60
44	53.03	34	24.18	69	42.06
44.5	53.41	34.5	24.36	69.5	42.21
45	54.53	35	24.89	70	42.67
45.5	54.86	35.5	25.07	70.5	42.82
46	55.83	36	25.60	71	43.28
46.5	56.18	36.5	25.78	71.5	43.43
47	57.22	37	26.31	72	43.89
47.5	57.57	37.5	26.49	72.5	44.04
48	58.62	38	27.02	73	44.50
48.5	58.97	38.5	27.20	73.5	44.65

TABLE 7   (continued) Body Fat Calculation—Women

Conversion Constants to Predict Percentage of Body Fat—Women

HIPS		ABDOMEN		HEIGHT	
(M1) Inches	Constant A	(M2) Inches	Constant B	(M3) Inches	Constant C
49	60.02	39	27.73	74	45.11
49.5	60.37	39.5	27.91	74.5	45.26
50	61.42	40	28.44	75	45.72
50.5	61.77	40.5	28.62	75.5	45.87
51	62.81	41	29.15	76	46.32
51.5	63.16	41.5	29.33	76.5	46.47
52	64.21	42	29.87	77	46.93
52.5	64.56	42.5	30.05	77.5	47.08
53	65.61	43	30.58	78	47.54
53.5	65.96	43.5	30.76	78.5	47.69
54	67.00	44	31.29	79	48.15
54.5	67.35	44.5	31.47	79.5	48.30
55	68.40	45	32.00	80	48.76
55.5	68.75	45.5	32.18	80.5	48.91
56	69.80	46	32.71	81	49.37
56.5	70.15	46.5	32.89	81.5	49.52
57	71.19	47	33.42	82	19.98
57.5	71.54	47.5	33.60	82.5	50.13
58	72.59	48	34.13	83	50.59
58.5	72.94	48.5	34.31	83.5	50.74
59	73.99	49	34.84	84	51.20
59.5	74.34	49.5	35.02	84.5	51.35
60	75.39	50	35.56	85	51.81

TABLE 8 BODY FAT CALCULATION—MEN

(M3) Waist Minus Wrist (in inches)

(M4) Weight in pounds

Weight	22	22.5	23	23.5	24	24.5	25	25.5	26	26.5	27	27.5	28	28.5	29	29.5	30	30.5	31
120	4	6	8	10	12	14	16	18	20	21	23	25	27	29	31	33	35	37	39
125	4	6	7	9	11	13	15	17	19	20	22	24	26	28	30	32	33	35	37
130	3	5	7	9	11	12	14	16	18	20	21	23	25	27	28	30	32	34	36
135	3	5	7	8	10	12	13	15	17	19	20	22	24	26	27	29	31	32	34
140	3	5	6	8	10	11	13	15	16	18	19	21	23	24	26	28	29	31	33
145	3	4	6	7	9	11	12	14	15	17	19	20	22	23	25	27	28	30	31
150	2	4	6	7	9	10	12	13	15	16	18	19	21	23	24	26	27	29	30
155	2	4	5	6	8	10	11	13	14	16	17	19	20	22	23	25	26	28	29
160	2	4	5	6	8	9	11	12	14	15	17	18	20	21	22	24	25	27	28
165	2	3	5	6	8	9	10	12	13	15	16	17	19	20	22	23	24	26	27
170	2	3	4	6	7	9	10	11	13	14	15	17	18	19	21	22	24	25	26
175	2	3	4	6	7	8	10	11	12	13	15	16	17	19	20	21	23	24	25
180	1	3	4	5	7	8	9	10	12	13	14	16	17	18	19	21	22	23	25
185	1	3	4	5	6	8	9	10	11	13	14	15	16	18	19	20	21	22	24
190	1	2	4	5	6	7	8	9	11	12	13	15	16	17	18	19	21	22	23
195	1	2	3	5	6	7	8	9	11	12	13	14	15	16	18	19	20	2	22
200	1	2	3	4	6	7	8	9	10	11	12	14	15	16	17	18	19	2	22

(M3) Waist Minus Wrist (in inches)

(M4) Weight in pounds

	22	22.5	23	23.5	24	24.5	25	25.5	26	26.5	27	27.5	28	28.5	29	29.5	30	30.5	31
205	1	2	3	4	5	6	8	9	10	11	12	13	14	15	17	18	19	20	21
210	1	2	3	4	5	6	7	8	9	11	12	13	14	15	16	17	18	19	21
215	1	2	3	4	5	6	7	8	9	10	11	12	13	15	16	17	18	19	20
220	0	2	3	4	5	6	7	8	9	10	11	12	13	14	15	16	17	18	19
225	0	1	2	3	4	6	7	8	9	10	11	12	13	14	15	16	17	18	19
230	0	1	2	3	4	5	6	7	8	9	10	11	12	13	14	15	16	17	18
235	0	1	2	3	4	5	6	7	8	9	10	11	12	13	14	15	16	17	18
240	0	1	2	3	4	5	6	7	8	9	10	11	12	13	14	15	16	17	17
245	0	1	2	3	4	5	6	7	8	9	9	10	11	12	13	14	15	16	17
250	0	1	2	3	4	5	6	6	7	8	9	10	11	12	13	14	15	16	16
255	0	1	2	3	4	5	5	6	7	8	9	10	11	12	13	14	14	15	16
260	0	1	2	2	3	4	5	6	7	8	9	9	10	11	12	13	14	15	15
265	0	—	1	2	3	4	5	6	7	8	8	9	10	11	12	13	14	14	15
270	0	—	1	2	3	4	5	6	7	8	8	9	10	11	12	13	13	14	15
275	0	0	1	2	3	4	5	5	6	7	8	9	10	11	11	12	13	14	14
280	0	0	1	2	3	4	4	5	6	7	8	9	9	10	11	12	13	14	14
285	0	0	1	2	3	4	4	5	6	7	8	8	9	10	11	12	12	13	14
290	0	0	1	2	3	4	4	5	6	7	7	8	9	10	11	11	12	13	14
295	0	0	1	2	3	4	4	5	6	6	7	8	9	10	10	11	12	13	14
300	0	0	1	2	3	3	4	5	5	6	7	8	9	9	10	11	12	12	13

(continued)

TABLE 8 *(continued)* Body Fat Calculation—Men

(M3) Waist Minus Wrist (in inches)

(M4) Weight in pounds

Weight	31.5	32	32.5	33	33.5	34	34.5	35	35.5	36	36.5	37	37.5	38	38.5	39	39.5	40	40.5
120	41	43	45	47	49	50	52	54	56	58	60	62	64	66	68	70	70	74	76
125	39	41	43	45	46	48	50	52	54	56	58	59	61	63	65	67	69	71	72
130	37	39	41	43	44	46	48	50	52	53	55	57	59	61	62	64	66	68	69
135	36	38	39	41	43	44	46	48	50	51	53	55	56	58	60	62	63	65	67
140	34	36	38	39	41	43	44	46	48	49	51	53	54	56	58	59	61	63	64
145	33	35	36	38	39	41	43	44	46	47	49	51	52	54	55	57	59	60	62
150	32	33	35	36	38	40	41	43	44	46	47	49	50	52	53	55	57	58	60
155	31	32	34	35	37	38	40	41	43	44	46	47	49	50	52	53	55	56	58
160	30	31	33	34	35	37	38	40	41	43	44	46	47	48	50	51	53	54	56
165	29	30	31	33	34	36	37	38	40	41	43	44	45	47	48	50	51	52	54
170	28	29	30	32	33	34	36	37	39	40	41	43	44	45	47	48	49	51	52
175	27	28	29	31	32	33	35	36	37	39	40	41	43	44	45	47	48	49	51
180	26	27	28	30	31	32	34	35	36	37	39	40	41	43	44	45	47	48	49
185	25	26	28	29	30	31	33	34	35	36	38	39	40	41	43	44	45	46	48
190	24	26	27	28	29	30	32	33	34	35	37	38	39	40	41	43	44	45	46
195	24	25	26	27	28	30	31	32	33	34	35	37	38	39	40	41	43	44	45
200	23	24	25	26	28	29	30	31	32	33	35	36	37	38	39	40	41	43	44

(M3) Waist Minus Wrist (in inches)																		
31.5	32	32.5	33	33.5	34	34.5	35	35.5	36	36.5	37	37.5	38	38.5	39	39.5	40	40.5
(M4) Weight in pounds																		
205	22	23	25	26	27	28	29	30	31	32	34	35	36	37	38	39	40	41	43
210	22	23	24	25	26	27	28	29	30	32	33	34	35	36	37	38	39	40	42
215	21	22	23	24	25	26	28	29	30	31	32	33	34	35	36	37	38	39	40
220	20	22	23	24	25	26	27	28	29	30	31	32	33	34	35	36	37	38	39
225	20	21	22	23	24	25	26	27	28	29	30	31	32	33	34	35	36	37	38
230	19	20	21	22	23	24	25	26	27	28	30	31	32	33	34	35	36	37	38
235	19	20	21	22	23	24	25	26	27	28	29	30	31	32	33	34	35	36	37
240	18	19	20	21	22	23	24	25	26	27	28	29	30	31	32	33	34	35	36
245	18	19	20	21	22	23	24	25	26	27	27	28	29	30	31	32	33	34	35
250	18	18	19	20	21	22	23	24	25	26	27	28	29	30	31	31	32	33	34
255	17	18	19	20	21	22	23	24	24	25	26	27	28	29	30	31	32	33	34
260	17	17	19	19	20	21	22	23	24	25	26	27	27	28	29	30	31	32	33
265	16	17	18	19	20	21	22	22	23	24	25	26	27	28	29	29	30	31	32
270	16	16	18	19	19	20	21	22	23	24	25	25	26	27	28	29	30	31	31
275	16	16	17	18	19	20	21	22	22	23	24	25	26	27	27	28	29	30	31
280	15	16	17	17	19	19	20	21	22	23	24	24	25	26	27	28	29	29	30
285	15	16	17	17	18	19	20	21	21	22	23	24	25	26	26	27	28	29	30
290	15	15	16	17	18	19	19	20	21	22	23	23	24	25	26	27	27	28	29
295	14	15	16	17	17	18	19	20	21	21	22	23	24	25	25	26	27	28	28
300	14	15	16	16	17	18	19	19	20	21	22	22	23	24	25	26	26	27	28

(continued)

TABLE 8 (continued) Body Fat Calculation—Men

(M3) Waist Minus Wrist (in inches)

(M4) Weight in pounds

	41	41.5	42	42.5	43	43.5	44	44.5	45	45.5	46	46.5	47	47.5	48	48.5	49	49.5	50
120	77	79	81	83	85	87	89	91	93	95	97	99	99	99	99	99	99	99	99
125	74	76	78	80	82	84	85	87	89	91	93	95	96	98	99	99	99	99	99
130	71	73	75	77	78	80	82	84	86	87	89	91	93	94	96	98	99	99	99
135	68	70	72	74	75	77	79	80	82	84	86	87	89	91	92	94	96	98	99
140	66	68	69	71	72	74	76	77	79	81	82	84	86	87	89	91	92	94	96
145	63	65	67	68	70	71	73	75	76	78	79	81	83	84	86	87	89	91	92
150	61	63	64	66	67	69	70	72	74	75	77	78	80	81	83	84	86	87	89
155	59	61	62	64	65	67	68	70	71	73	74	76	77	79	80	82	83	85	86
160	57	59	60	61	63	64	66	67	69	70	72	73	75	76	77	79	80	82	83
165	55	57	58	60	61	62	64	65	67	68	69	71	72	74	75	75	78	79	81
170	54	55	56	58	59	60	62	63	64	66	67	69	70	71	73	74	75	77	78
175	52	53	55	56	57	59	61	61	63	64	65	66	68	69	70	72	73	74	76
180	50	52	53	54	56	57	58	59	61	62	63	65	66	67	68	70	71	72	74
185	49	50	51	53	54	55	56	58	59	60	61	63	64	65	66	63	69	70	71
190	48	49	50	51	52	54	55	56	57	58	60	61	62	63	65	65	67	68	69
195	46	47	49	50	51	52	53	55	56	57	58	59	60	62	63	64	65	66	68
200	45	46	47	48	50	51	52	53	54	55	57	58	59	60	61	62	63	65	66

•→ Appendix 2 ←•

Sex-Busting Drugs

The following commonly prescribed drugs have been linked to erectile dysfunction and loss of libido. The brand-name drug products associated with these problems number in the hundreds. If a medication that you are using falls into one of these broad categories but you cannot find it among the examples below, consult your physician.

Antidepressants

If you are taking any of the following drugs, it may be the cause of your sexual problems.

Elavil (amitriptyline)
Pamelor (nortriptline)
Prozac (fluoxetine)
Zoloft (sertraline)

Blood Pressure and Cardiovascular Medications

If you are taking one of the following drugs or another antihypertensive drug, it could be the source of your trouble.

Beta andrenergic blockers
Calan (verapamil)
Calcium channel blockers
Catapres (clonidine)
Diuretics

HydroDIURIL (hydrochlorothiazide)
Inderal (propranolol)
Tenormin (atenolol)

Antihistamines

These drugs can cause sexual dysfunction as well as drowsiness and fatigue.

Allegra (fexofenadine)
Benadryl (diphenhydramine)
Claritin (loratadine)
Dramamine (dimenhydrinate)

Anti-Ulcer Drugs

Histamine-2 receptor blocking drugs have been strongly linked to sexual problems.

Tagamet (cimetidine)
Zantac (ranitidine hydrochloride)

Proscar / Propecia (Finasteride)

This drug is highly prescribed to prevent both hair loss and prostate growth. It is linked both to erectile dysfunction and loss of libido.

·← Appendix 3 →·

Exercise

Use this appendix to supplement Chapters 4, 5, 7, and 8. The information is divided into three main types of exercise described in the book: fat loss, muscle building, and pro-sexual.

Fat Loss Exercise

The old-fashioned concept of exercise is that only aerobic exercise is necessary for maintaining weight loss and decreasing fat levels. The new concept is that two types of exercise—aerobic and anaerobic—are needed for weight management and maximum health. Recent studies have shown that even though in the short term the same amount of calories can be burned by either aerobic exercise alone or a mixture of aerobic and anaerobic exercise, over the long run more fat-weight loss is gained if both are used.

Aerobic exercise refers to the process of aerobic (with oxygen) burning of sugar-glucose and other fuels (amino acids, fats). Aerobic capacity is the ability of your cardiopulmonary system to deliver blood and oxygen to active muscles. It also determines the capacity of these muscles to use oxygen and fuel (glucose, fat, amino acids) to perform exercise or physical work.

Anaerobic exercise (without oxygen) involves using glucose only as a fuel, with energy production occurring without the presence of oxygen. That is why most of us can't maintain it long. An example is dashing up three flights of stairs as fast as you can. The anaerobic form of energy production is a short-term system dependent on the stores of sugar-glycogen in your muscle or liver. Since oxygen is not initially used, eventually you develop an oxygen debt that you pay by "being winded" and having to "catch" your breath later on.

Lactic acid is a by-product of anaerobic exercise. It can produce a

burning sensation in your muscles. If strenuous anaerobic exercise continues long enough (usually no more than two to three minutes is possible for a thirty-five- to fifty-five-year-old), you can "hit the wall" and
have to quit or drop from exhaustion. That's because energy production cannot keep up with energy demands and the resultant lactic acid
buildup. Your anaerobic capacity can be determined by a blood lactic
acid level measured in an exercise physiology laboratory during maximal exercise on a treadmill.

If you are out of shape or fat, your body cannot handle anaerobic exercise as well as your more fit peers. (Similarly, older persons on the average cannot sustain anaerobic exercise as well as their younger
counterparts, but of course this is highly dependent on the level of fitness.) Your system does not produce energy anaerobically as well, and
the lactic acid you make cannot be eliminated as quickly from the body.
However, with proper training you can regain much of this lost capacity, and, best of all, these gains can be made at virtually any age. So,
baby boomers and young seniors, there are no excuses for not becoming more fit!

How can you determine if you are exercising aerobically (with oxygen) or anaerobically (without oxygen)? Most exercise trainers calculate an ideal anaerobic-aerobic target heart rate by using this formula:

1. Determine your maximum heart rate: Subtract your age from 220.
   For example, your maximum heart rate is 180 if you are forty
   years old. This is probably the maximum heart rate you can attain
   at your age with strenuous exercise.
2. Determine your cardiovascular condition: Select the percentage of
   maximum heart rate for sustained exercise from the list below that
   best describes your current fitness level. (Be brutally honest!)

   • Out of Shape: You have a sedentary lifestyle and do little if any
     exercise. You're probably overweight, flabby, or both. If this describes you, begin exercising at 50 to 60 percent of your maximum heart rate. Using the example above, if 180 is your target
     heart rate, then your goal is 90 to 108 beats per minute. You
     should be able to train at this heart rate aerobically. Going
     above this heart rate may put you into "oxygen debt" (anaerobic) exercise training, and you may start to get winded.

•→ *Caution:* Persons very overweight or obese (fifteen pounds or
    more) should consult their physician before beginning any type of
    exercise program.

- Moderate to Good Shape: You have a fairly active lifestyle and get at least some sustained exercise on a weekly basis. You are not overweight or are less than five pounds above your ideal weight. If this describes you, continue exercising at 65 to 70 percent of your maximum heart rate. Using the example above, if 180 is your target heart rate, then your goal is 117 to 126 beats per minute. You should be able to train at this heart rate aerobically. Going above this heart rate may put you into "oxygen debt" (anaerobic) exercise training, and you may start to get winded.
- Very Good Shape: You have an active lifestyle in which you exercise at least three times a week. If this describes you, try exercising at 75 percent of your maximum heart rate to maximize your workouts. Using the above example, if 180 is your target rate, then your goal is 135 beats per minute. You should be able to train at this heart rate aerobically. Going above this heart rate may put you into "oxygen debt" (anaerobic) exercise training, and you may start to get winded.

A quick way to tell which exercise mode you are in is the simple talking test: Can you talk and exercise at the same time? If you are able to talk and exercise and not be out of breath, then you are in an aerobic mode. If you are unable to talk and exercise at the same time because you are out of breath, then you are in an anaerobic mode. Here are some examples of each:

Low-Intensity Aerobic Exercise

1. Stroll on a flat surface with a dog or young children.
2. Pedal an exercise bike with no resistance.
3. Lift light weights over and over with no strain and not get out of breath.
4. Mow the lawn or rake leaves at an easy pace.

Intense Anaerobic Exercise Examples

1. Run up two to six flights of stairs as fast as you can without stopping.
2. Sprint as fast as you can for one to two minutes.
3. Walk up a steep hill as fast as you can.
4. Use an exercise bike against a lot of resistance.

For effective fat loss, your program should include both aerobic and anaerobic exercise. I recommend a ratio of fifteen seconds to one minute of anaerobic (out-of-breath mode) exercise for every ten to fifteen minutes of aerobic exercise. See what works best for you and keep a log to help monitor your progress. But keep your exercise regimen mixed to train all parts of your body's energy-producing machinery and to maximize your metabolism.

Muscle-Building Exercise

In Chapter 5 you learned how a weight-training program can be used in conjunction with T-boosters to build muscle mass. If you have never used weights before, consult a professionally licensed personal or exercise trainer. He or she can show you proper technique for lifting weights, which is important to know in order to avoid overstraining and incurring injuries. The initial one-time consultation fee is an investment that will reap you rewards for the rest of your life. If you already belong to a gym, chances are there is a qualified exercise trainer on staff who can assist you.

The program that a trainer designs for you should work different parts of the body on different days. A weekly regimen of weight training might look like the following:

- Mondays: Focus on strengthening the middle section of the body and back, working muscles of the trunk and abdomen.
- Wednesdays: Focus on the lower body and the quadriceps muscles of the leg. Exercises include the machine quad extension and the machine standing calf extension.
- Fridays or Saturdays: Focus on the upper body and muscles of the shoulders, back, arms, and chest.

Here are the basic rules of weight training we use at our Sports Medicine and Anti-Aging Clinic in Santa Monica, California:

1. Do not weight-train for more than twenty-five to forty minutes in one day; otherwise, you can overtrain and cause a decline in your natural anabolic hormones. That will defeat the purpose of your program and increase oxidative (free radicals) stress.
2. Do not use weights more than two days in a row. Continuous daily training can slow down the muscle-building process.

3. Always begin your weight-training session first with twenty minutes or so of aerobic exercise (enough to get you sweating) so that when the weights are started, your tissues are warm and pliable and less likely to be injured.

4. Do two sets of each type of weight-resistance exercise. First set: ten to fifteen repetitions. Second set: six to eight repetitions with an increased weight. When you are at the last two or three repetitions, you should have a feeling of muscle "failure." If you don't, then the weight needs to be increased. The total number of sets per training session should be limited to a maximum of nine to twelve.

5. Identify your starting lift (first-set weight) with the one-lift maximum test. Find the maximum weight with which you can do only one lift. Start light and work up, or have your trainer assist you with the help of a chart that can determine your maximum one lift. Start by using a weight that is 60 percent to 70 percent of that maximum weight. That's the starting weight for your first set. Example: If you can lift only forty pounds once and no more, then your initial lift weight is about twenty-five to thirty pounds.

6. Increase your initial weight until you can do six or eight repetitions. That is your second set lift.

7. After two sets, move on to the next weight-resistance exercise.

8. After a weight-training session, stretch out the areas just exercised and any other tight muscles for at least forty-five seconds to one minute per stretch A stretch doesn't work unless it is held at least that long.

Pro-Sexual Exercise

To maximize pleasure and performance, the body's sexual energy system must be in balance. In Chapter 7 you determined your sexual nature from the yin-yang sexual mode questionnaire. If your score was not where you would like it to be, you can balance and improve your sexuality with these time-tested yogic exercises. Depending on your score, follow either the yin or yang pro-sexual exercise program.

Yin

Your moderate to high yin sexual mode score indicates that you are sexually and physically lacking in sexual energy. Your internal system is excessively expanded, cool, and asexual. Indeed, you may have decided to join the ranks of the celibate because you have lost or are slowly losing your sexual heat—that is, your androgenic yang sexual energy.

In the world of yoga, the body's heat source comes from the energy center called the solar plexus, also known as the "seat of physical energy," the third chakra, or Manipura (which translates into "place of the jewel" or "lotus of the navel"). The erotic stirs up the heat or fire of love, which consists of four types: habitual, natural, imaginary, and sensual. Most love is a blend of the four types. Sensual love is heightened by stimulating the three physical energy points, or chakras, connected with sexuality.

The first chakra lies above the anus, just below the base of the penis, or one to two inches below the vaginal opening. The second chakra is located above the pubic bone area over the bladder. The third chakra—the navel—is where all physical sexuality starts.

These exercises are designed to increase sexual heat by stimulating the third chakra, which in turn stimulates the first and second. The heat you generate will help with the firing of your sexual nerves. This, in turn, will build better erections, vaginal lubrication, labial and clitoral swelling, heightened sexual sensitivity, sexual contractions, and orgasms.

Solar Plexus Squeeze
Concentrate on stimulating and building the fire in the solar plexus. Visualize a fire of hot sexual energy moving down from the solar plexus (under the navel) to above the pubic bone and then down to the base of the spine. When you feel the energy has moved there, look down slightly and squeeze your buttocks together for ten seconds and repeat ten times. Repeat this exercise four times daily. The exercise can be performed anytime you are sitting—for example, while at your desk.

You should feel a little heat in your face when performing the exercise properly. If not, then squeeze your buttocks a little harder. You can also do this standing, but only with a good erect posture, with the chest out and the chin in.

Seated Solar Plexus Stomach Lift
Sit in a chair or on the floor with an erect spine and with your chest out. Take a big breath, then completely exhale. Swallow and pull in your stomach—the abdomen and the navel—as far as you can toward your spinal column.

Focus your attention on the flow of sexual heat from the navel down to the bladder area and then to your loins. Keep it at the base of the spine. Squeeze the buttocks tightly and hold for ten to fifteen seconds, then exhale. Repeat the exercise three to six times or more, three times daily.

Standing Solar Plexus Stomach Lift
Stand with your feet apart, knees slightly bent, and hands on the corresponding knees. As you exhale and completely empty the lungs, tighten the abdomen muscles to form a hollow. Gradually release the abdomen and inhale slowly. Repeat the exercise three to seven times or more, three times daily.

Solar Plexus Bellows
Sit on the floor erect, with your feet crossed and your wrists resting on your knees. Look at your navel and at the tip of your nose at the same time. Take in a deep breath through the nose. Hold for three to four seconds, then exhale completely. Swallow and draw your navel back and forth as many times as possible. Stop if you are tired or dizzy. Do not hurry; quality is better than quantity. Each day try to do one or two more than the day before.

•➤ *Caution:* Do these exercises only on an empty stomach. Avoid these exercises if you have any nerve problems in your spine, pain down the legs, numbness or tingling down the legs, or high blood pressure that is not controlled.

Yang

Your moderate to high yang sexual mode score indicates that you need to cool down your sexual energy.

The purpose of these exercises is to dampen the excessive fire in the first three chakras—the belly, the loins, and the groin. This is the path of celibacy. Use it to the degree needed to control hypersexual behavior and thoughts. In general, think of the process of transmuting your overly heightened sexuality into other forms of energy—the higher mental faculties. Yogis typically practice breathing exercises four times a day to keep their sexual thoughts under control.

Flat Back
Lie flat on your back, arms at sides, palms facing upward, and feet relaxed with no pointed toes. Breathe normally and relax in this pose for two minutes. The objective is to extinguish excessive heat in your body. Visualize that you are super-hot and now all the tension-heat in your

body is being released, like water evaporating. With each breath your body is getting lighter, floating weightless as in a spaceship with no gravity.

Prayer Stretch
Kneel with your buttocks resting on your heels. As you exhale slowly, bend slowly forward until the palms of your hands and your forehead touch the floor. There should be a straight line from your tailbone to your fingertips. Hold the position and stretch the spine. (If your knees or shoulders hurt, stretch to the point of comfort.) Feel the release of tension. As you breathe normally, relax the buttocks and let the heat dissipate from the pelvic area. Visualize coolness and calmness. Concentrate on the point between the eyebrows and visualize all sexual impulses being transformed into cosmic joy, unity, and love with no physical attachments. Hold this pose for at least fifteen seconds. Repeat this exercise as needed.

Plow Pose
Lie flat on your back with hands alongside the body and palms against the floor. As you hold your breath, slowly raise your legs without bending your knees. When your legs are at a 90-degree angle, raise your hips and the lower part of your back. While gradually exhaling, lower legs over the head as far as is comfortable. (The objective is to have the toes touch the floor behind the head.) Visualize sexual urges, impulses, and heat being discharged from the base of the spine and down from the backs of the thighs and out through the toes.

If you feel pain or numbness down the legs, then stop or do the exercise only to a pain-free point. Hold the exercise for a few seconds, then try to go farther toward the ground with the toes again. Over time you will be able to go farther and longer, but always use comfort as your guide.

•➤ *Caution:* Stop if you get dizzy. Avoid this exercise if you have any problems with the blood vessels from the neck into the head or if you have back or neck problems.

⋆ Appendix 4 ⋆

Supplement Suppliers

The following companies sell T-booster products. While they are known to be reputable, this listing does not constitute an endorsement.

Genetic Evolutionary Nutrition
Unit 7
4040 Del Rey Avenue
Del Rey, CA 90292
(310) 301-4979; toll free (800) 414-4366
Fax (310) 301-8041
www.genn.com
GEN was one of the first companies to sell prohormones. They now sell almost every prohormone as well as tribulus and chrysin. GEN also carries many other sports nutrition and antiaging supplements.

LPJ Reasearch Products
205 South Main Street
P.O. Box 227
Seymour, IL 61875
(217) 687-4455
Fax (217) 687-4830
E-mail: parnold_8@ix.netcom.com
Patrick Arnold's company developed many of the new generation of T-booster products and offers an advanced supplement line for sale directly to the public.

Mesomorphosis Inc.
Suite 103
14209 Cyber Place
Tampa, FL 33613-2788
(813) 972-8991
Fax (813) 972-2688
www.mesomorphosis.com

This Internet site sells several different brands of prohormones as well as many other sports nutrition supplements and books. Also includes numerous articles and information about prohormones.

Metabolic Response Modifiers
2633 W. Pacific Coast Highway, Suite B
Newport Beach, CA 92663
(800) 948-6296
E-mail: sales@metabolicresponse.com
www.metamode.com
Carries many prohormone products. The company invests a portion of its net profits into research, and has funded some studies on prohormones.

Nutritional Experience
11670 National Boulevard, #213
Los Angeles, CA 90064
(310) 716-8549
(310) 391-1829
www.nutritionalexperience.com
An Internet-based company run by Los Angeles nutritionist Mason Panetti, Nutritional Experience includes a wide range of prohormones and other sports nutrition and antiaging products.

Nutritional Warehouse
405 South Lincoln Boulevard
Venice, CA 90291
(301) 392-3636
E-mail: Nutritionwaveh@WebTV.net

Olympia Nutrition
3579 Highway 50 East, #220
Carson City, NV 89701
(888) 366-9909
Fax (800) 877-3292
www.smart-drugs.com/olymprod.html
E-mail: olympia@smart-drugs.com
Olympia Nutrition is a mail order supplement company specializing in antiaging supplements. It sells several prohormone products as well as many antioxidants and other supplements intended to prevent and reverse the symptoms of aging.

Osmo Therapy
2471 American Avenue
Hayward, CA 94545
(510) 265-2445
The first supplement company to sell prohormones, Osmo Therapy introduced androstenedione under the trade name Androstene 50 in 1997. They now offer a line of several prohormone products as well as other bodybuilding and sports nutrition products.

Substrate Solutions
2112 Business Center Drive
Irvine, CA 92612
(949) 622-0500
www.substratesolutions.com
A subsidiary of the major sports nutrition company Met-Rx, Substrate Solutions offers a full line of prohormone products, including nor-4-adiol (sold under the brand name Norandrodiol).

⤙ Glossary ⤚

Acetyl-L-Carnitine (ALC): a quasi-amino acid that occurs naturally in the body, where it plays a role in the transport of fats into the mitochondria and in the formation of neurotransmitters in the brain.

Acupressure: a type of massage therapy using finger pressure on the bodily sites used in acupuncture.

Adenosine Triphosphate (ATP): a high-energy molecule that is the primary source of energy in all living cells because of its function in donating a phosphate group during biochemical activities.

Adrenal Gland: one of a pair of ductless organs, located above the kidneys, consisting of a cortex, which produces steroidal hormones, and a medulla, which produces epinephrine and norepinephrine.

Alzheimer's Disease: a pathological exaggeration of aging disease that shows drastic failure of cognitive ability, loss of memory and orientation, and progressive decline in intellectual functioning; shows cortical atrophy and reduction of metabolism in the brain's posterior parietal cortex and temporal lobe.

Amygdala: a brain structure of the limbic system that is involved in emotions of fear and aggression.

Anabolic Androgenic Steroid (AAS): a class of steroid hormone, especially testosterone, that promotes growth of muscle tissue.

Androgen: a substance, such as testosterone or dihydrotestosterone, that promotes male characteristics.

Androstenedione (Adione): a sex hormone that is a direct precursor to testosterone and estrogen.

Antagonize: to act in opposition.

Antidepressant: a drug used to relieve or treat mental depression.

Arginine: an essential free amino acid that may increase blood vessel dilation.

Beta Sitosterol: a plant extract that has similar structure to steroid hormones, such as testosterone and estrogen.

Biochemistry: the scientific study of the chemical substances and processes of living matter.

Biopsy: the removal for diagnostic study of a piece of tissue from a living body.

Boron: a nonmetallic element occurring naturally only in combination, as in borax or boric acid; may increase sex hormone levels in postmenopausal women.

Calorie: a unit defining the heat output of an organism and the energy value of food.

Carbohydrate: any of a class of organic compounds composed of carbon, hydrogen, and oxygen, including starches and sugars; produced in green plants by photosynthesis; important food source for people.

Castrate: to remove the testes or ovaries.

Cholesterol: a steroid molecule that functions in the body as a membrane constituent and as a precursor of steroid hormones and bile acids.

Chrysin: an herbal supplement touted to increase the levels of testosterone in the body.

Cimetidine: an anti-ulcer drug; its trade name is Tagamet.

Cognitive Disorder: malfunction in the mental processes of perception, memory, judgment, and reasoning, as contrasted with emotional and volitional processes.

Cortisol: one of several steroid hormones produced by the adrenal cortex and resembling cortisone in its action; induces muscle and other tissue breakdown.

Creatine Monohydrate: an amino acid that is a constituent of the muscles of vertebrates and is combined with phosphoric acid or a phosphorus-containing group in order to store energy used for muscular contraction.

Creatine Phosphate: a molecule that allows the body to regenerate the energy-producing molecule called ATP.

Creatinine: a protein breakdown product that is excreted by the kidneys.

Damiana: an herb that contains beta sitosterol and other compounds that produce a mild stimulatory effect.

DHEA: dehydroepiandrosterone, a steroid hormone naturally produced by the adrenal glands and sold in synthetic form as a nutritional supplement to raise testosterone and estrogen levels.

Dopamine: a monoamine neurotransmitter that acts within certain brain cells to help regulate movement, emotions, and sexual energy.

Endocrinology: the study of the endocrine glands and their secretions, especially in relation to their processes or functions.

Ego: the conscious, rational component of the psyche that experiences and reacts to the outside world and mediates between the demands of the id and the superego.

Erectile: capable of being distended with blood and becoming rigid of tissue.

Estrogen: any of several major female sex hormones produced primarily by ovarian folllicles that are capable of inducing estrus, producing secondary female sex characteristics, and preparing the uterus for the reception of a fertilized egg.

4-Androstenediol (4-adiol): a hormone that occurs in small quantities in the human body and is a direct precursor to testosterone.

5-Androstenediol (5-adiol): a hormone that can either convert to testosterone or convert to DHEA in the human body.

Ginkgo Biloba: the oldest living tree species from which extracts are made and sold for a wide variety of uses.

Ginseng: any plant of the genus *Panax* having an aromatic root used medicinally throughout Asia; it is prepared as tea or as an extract made from the root.

Glutamine: a crystalline amino acid related to glutamic acid and found in many plant and animal proteins.

Glycemic Foods: substances that rapidly raise sugar and insulin blood levels when ingested.

High-Density Lipoprotein (HDL): a circulating combined form of lipid and protein that picks up cholesterol in the arteries and deposits it in the liver for reprocessing or excretion.

Hydrochloride: a salt, especially of an alkaloid, formed by the direct union of hydrochloric acid with an organic base.

Id: the part of the psyche that is the source of unconscious and instinctive impulses that seek satisfaction in accordance with the pleasure principle of Freud.

Immune System: a diffuse, complex network of interacting cells and cell products that protects the body from other foreign substances by destroying infection and malignant cells.

Ipriflavone: a drug sold in Hungary, Italy, and other coutnries that is used to increase bone mass and treat osteoporosis.

Kava kava: a shrub of the *Piper methysticum* pepper family whose roots are used to make an intoxicating beverage.

Labium: folds of skin bordering the external female genitalia.

Lactic Acid: product resulting from anaerobic metabolism in the body.

Libido: sexual instinct, energies, and desires that are derived from the id.

Lipoprotein: a lipid combined with a simple protein.

L-tryptophan: an essential amino acid used as an appetite suppressant and relaxant by promoting serotonin production.

Melatonin: a hormone secreted by the pineal gland in inverse proportion to the amount of light received by the retina; it is important in regulating bio-rhythms.

Metabolism: the sum of the physical and chemical processes in an organism by which its substance is produced, maintained, and destroyed, and by which energy is made available.

Metabolite: any substance derived from metabolism.

Methandriol: an injectable version of 5-androstenediol.

Muira Puama: an herb grown in the rain forest that contains beta sitosterol and other substances.

NADH: the reduced form of nicotinamide adenine dinucleotide (NAD), which plays a major role in electron transport reactions to create energy, adenosine triphosphate, and dopamine release.

Neurotransmitter: several chemical substances that send nerve impulse across a gap or junction.

Nocturnal Orgasm: spontaneous ejaculation during sleep.

Nor-androstenedione (Nor-Adione): a direct precursor to nor-testosterone.

Nor-5-Androstenediol (Nor-5-Adiol): a prohormone that converts to nor-testosterone in very small amounts.

Nor-4-Androstenediol (Nor-4-Adiol): a direct precursor to nor-testosterone.

Nor-testosterone: a hormone similar to testosterone with a high anabolic/androgenic ratio. Sold widely as an anabolic steroid.

Orgasm: the intense physical and emotional sensation experienced at the peak of sexual excitation.

Osteoporosis: a disease in which the bones become increasingly porous, brittle, and subject to fracture, from loss of calcium and other components.

Ovary: the female gonad or reproductive gland in which the ova and female sex hormones develop.

Over-the-counter (OTC): refers to any pharmaceutical item sold legally without a prescription, especially drugs.

Ovulation: production and discharge of eggs from an ovary or ovarian follicle.

Oxytocin: a pituitary hormone that stimulates contraction of the smooth muscles of the uterus during orgasm and to induce labor.

Pharmacology: the science that deals with the preparation, uses, and the effects of drugs.

Pheromone: any chemical substance released by an animal that serves to influence the physiology or behavior of other members of the same species.

Phosphatidylserine (PS): a lipid found in the brain that is vital for healthy neurological function. Found naturally in soybeans and is sold as a supplement.

Phytoestrogen: an estrogen-like substance found in specific plants.

Postmenopause: the period after the natural cessation of menstruation; it usually occurs between the age of fifty-two and fifty-five.

Precursors: a chemical that is transformed into another compound, as in the course of chemical reaction, and precedes that compound in the pathway.

Progesterone: a female hormone synthesized chiefly in the corpus luteum of the ovary; its function in the menstrual cycle is to prepare the uterus for a fertilized ovum.

Progestin: any substance that has activity similar to natural progesterone.

Prolactin: a pituitary hormone that stimulates milk production in mammals and lowers testosterone levels.

Prostate Gland: a partly muscular organ that surrounds the urethra of males at the base of the bladder and secretes an alkaline fluid that makes up part of the semen.

Protein: a molecule composed of twenty or more amino acids linked in one or more long chains; the final shape and properties of each protein are determined by the side chains of the amino acids and their chemical attachments.

Provera (Medroxyprogesterone): a synthetic drug similar to progesterone that is prescribed widely for postmenopausal women.

Prozac: a drug that inhibits the release of serotonin and is used chiefly as an antidepressant.

Psyllium: the seeds of the fleawort used as a mild laxative, especially in breakfast cereals.

Relaxant: a drug that induces a feeling of calm, especially one that lessens strain in a muscle or nervous system.

Saturated Fat: any animal or vegetable compound, abundant in fatty meats, dairy products, coconut oil, and palm oil, that tends to raise cholesterol levels in the blood.

Saw Palmetto: a shrublike palm, *Serenoa repens*, native to the southern United States and having green or blue leaf stalks set with spiny teeth. It is used to assist with prostate problems.

Sedative: a drug or agent used to allay irritability or excitement.

Serotonin: an amine that occurs in blood and nervous tissue and acts as a neurotransmitter in the brain.

7-Keto DHEA: a metabolite of DHEA that cannot convert to sex hormones.

Smilax: a plant of the lily family that grows in tropical and temperate zones, consisting mostly of woody-stemmed vines that contain beta sitosterol.

Starch: a white, tasteless, solid carbohydrate that is broken down rapidly by enzymes to form glucose, galactose, and fructose, important food elements.

Steroid. any of a large group of fat-soluble organic compounds, such as the sterols, bile acids, and sex hormones, most of which have specific physiological action.

Superego: the part of the personality representing the conscience, formed in early life by the internalization of the standards of parents and other models of behavior.

T-Boosters: also known as testosterone prohormones since they convert testosterone or nor-testosterone in the human body via chemical reaction.

Testosterone: the hormone that stimulates the development of male sex organs, secondary sexual male traits, and sperm.

Thermogenics: supplements that cause the body's temperature to rise.

Thyroid: a gland situated in the lower part of the front of the neck that secretes a hormone that plays a major role in regulating the metabolic rate of other tissues of the body.

Thyroxine (T-4): a hormone of the thyroid gland that regulates the metabolic rate of the body.

Tranquilizer: any of various drugs, such as the benzodiazepines, that have a sedative, calming, or muscle-relaxing effect.

Transdermal: a medication applied to the skin for absorption into the bloodstream.

Transrectal Ultrasound Exam: a medical inspection of the prostate gland to detect prostate abnormalities.

Tribulus Terrestris: an ancient Indian herb that is sold and marketed as a drug by a Bulgarian pharmaceutical company.

Tricep: the muscle at the back of the upper arm.

Tyrosine: an amino acid that acts as a precursor of norepinephrine and dopamine, helps to increase brain levels of the neurotransmitter dopamine, which is essential for libido.

Urologist: a physician who specializes in diseases of the genitourinary tract.

Vaginal Atrophy: a wasting away of the vagina, as from deficient sex hormones or nerve damage.

Valium: a brand of diazepam, a benzodiazepine, used chiefly as a muscle relaxant and to alleviate anxiety.

Vasopressin: a hormone released by the posterior pituitary gland.

Vitamin: any group of organic substances essential to normal metabolism; found in minute amounts in natural foodstuff and also produced synthetically. Deficiencies in vitamins produce specific disorders.

Yohimbé: a tropical West African tree extract (*Corynanthe yohimbe*) that yields an alkaloid promoted as an aphrodisiac.

Yohimbine Hydrochloride: a prescription formed with yohimbé to enhance blood circulation.

Zinc: a mineral essential for testosterone production and immune and antiviral function.

⋆⊷ Bibliography ⊷⋆

Chapter 1: The Dawn of the T-Booster Era

Becker, K.L. *Principles and Practice of Endocrinology and Metabolism.* Philadelphia, PA: J. B. Lippincott, 1990.

Bhasin, S., et al. "The Effects of Supraphysiologic Doses of Testosterone on Muscle Size and Strength in Normal Men." *New England Journal of Medicine* 335, no.1 (July 1996): 1–7.

Hill, Aubrey. *The Testosterone Solution.* Rocklin, CA: Prima Publishing, 1997.

Kalmijn, S., et al. "A Prospective Study on Cortisol, Dehydroepiandrosterone Sulfate, and Cognitive Function in the Elderly." *Journal of Clinical Endocrinology and Metabolism* 83, no. 10 (1998): 3487–92.

Labrie, Fernand, et. al., "Physiological Changes in Dehydroepiandrosterone Are Not Reflected by Serum Levels of Active Androgens but of Their Metabolites: Intracrinology." *Journal of Clinical Endocrinology and Metabolism* 82, no. 8 (1997): 2403–09.

Taniguchi, N., and Kaneko, S. "Alcoholic Effect on Male Sexual Function." *Nippon Rinsho* 55, no. 11 (1997): 3040–44.

Taylor, William N. *Macho Medicine: A History of the Anabolic Steroid Epidemic.* Jefferson, NC: McFarland Press, 1991.

Ullis, Karlis, and Ptacek, Greg. *Age Right: Turn Back the Clock with a Proven, Personalized Antiaging Program.* New York: Simon & Schuster, 1999.

Wadler, G. I., and Hainline, B. *Drugs and the Athlete.* Philadelphia, PA: F. A. Davis, 1989.

Chapter 2: The First Generation of Sex Enhancers

Bidzinska, B., et al. "Effects of Different Chronic Intermittent Stressors and Acetyl-L-Carnitine on Hypothalamic Beta-Endorphin and GnRH and on Plasma Testosterone in Rats." *Neuroendocrinology* 57 (1993): 985–90.

Choi, H. K., et al. "Clinical Efficacy of Korean Red Ginseng for Erectile Dysfunction." *International Journal of Impotence Research* 7, no. 3 (1995): 181–86.

Cogan, Michael. *Optimum Sports Nutrition: Your Competitive Edge.* New York: Advanced Research Press, 1993.

DeSilverio, F., et al. "Evidence That Serenoa Repens Extract Displays an Antiestrogenic Activity in Prostatic Tissue of Benign Prostatic Hypertrophy Patients." *European Urology* 21 (1992): 309–14.

Gennazani, A. D., et al. "Acetyl-L-Carnitine as Possible Drug in the Treatment of Hypothalamic Amenorrhea." *Obstetrics and Gynecology of Scandinavia* 70, no. 6 (1991): 487–92.

Le Bars, et al. "A Placebo-Controlled, Double-Blind, Randomized Trial of an Extract of Ginkgo Biloba for Dementia." *Journal of the American Medical Association* 278 (1997): 1327–32.

Om, A., and Chung, K. "Dietary Zinc Deficiency Alters 5-Alpha Reduction and Aromatization of Testosterone and Androgen and Estrogen Receptors in Rat Liver." *Journal of Nutrition* 126, no. 4 (Apr. 1996): 842–48.

Paniagua, R., et al. "Zinc, Prolactin, Gonadotropin, and Androgen Levels in Uremic Men." *Archives of Andrology* 8, no. 4 (June 1982): 271–75.

Prasad, A., et al. "Zinc Status and Serum Testosterone Levels of Healthy Adults." *Nutrition* 12, no. 5 (May 1996): 344–48.

Sahelian, Ray. *DHEA: A Practical Guide.* Marina Del Rey, CA: Be Happier Press, 1996.

Santesson, Johan. "Johan's Guide to Aphrodisiacs." http://www.santesson.com/aphrodis/.

Schottner, M.; Gansser, D.; and Spiteller, G. "Lignans from the Roots of Urtica Dioica and Their Metabolites Bind to Human Sex Hormone Binding Globulin (SHBG)." *Planta Medicine* 63, no. 6 (Dec. 1997): 529–32.

Sikora, R., et al., "Ginkgo Biloba Extract in the Therapy of Erectile Dysfunction." *Journal of Urology* 141 (1989): 188A.

Waynberg J., "Aphrodisiacs: Contributions to the Clinical Evaluation of the Traditional Use of Ptychopetalum." The First International Congress on Ethnopharmacology, France, June 1990.

Chapter 3: The New Generation of T-Boosters and Sex Enhancers

Arreola, F.; Paniagua, R.; Herrera, J.; Diaz-Bensussen, S.; Mondragon, L.; Bermudez, J.; Perez, E.; and Villalpando, S. "Low

Plasma Zinc and Androgen in Insulin-Dependent Diabetes Mellitus," *Archives of Andrology* 16, no. 2 (1986): 151–54.

Arver, S.; Dobs, A. S.; Meikle, A. W.; Allen, R. P.; Sanders S. W.; and Mazer, N. A. "Improvement of Sexual Function in Testosterone Deficient Men Treated for 1 Year with A Permeation Enhanced Testosterone Transdermal System." *Journal of Urology* 155 (May 1996): 604–1608.

Bancroft, J., et al. "Androgens and Sexual Behaviour in Women Using Oral Contraceptives." *Clinical Endocrinology* 12, no. 4 (1980): 327–40.

Bhasin, S.; Storer, T.; Berman, N.; Callegari, C.; Clevenger, B.; Phillips, J.; Bunnell, T.; Tricker, R.; Shirazi, A.; and Casaburi, R. "The Effects of Supraphysiologic Doses of Testosterone on Muscle Size and Strength in Normal Men." *New England Journal of Medicine* 335, no. 1 (Jul. 1996): 1–7.

Bidzinska, B., et al. "Effects of Different Chronic Intermittent Stressors and Acetyl-L-Carnitine on Hypothalamic Beta-Endorphin and GnRH and on Plasma Testosterone in Rats." *Neuroendocrinology* 57 (1993): 985–90.

Blaquier, J., et al. "In Vitro Metabolism of Androgens in Whole Human Blood." *Acta Endocrinologica* 55 (1967): 697–704.

Dobs, Adrian; S., Hoover; Donald.R.; Chen, Min-Chi; and Allen, Richard. "Pharmacokinetic Characteristics, Efficacy, and Safety of Buccal Testosterone in Hypogonadal Males: A Pilot Study." *Journal of Clinical Endocrinology and Metabolism* 83, no. 1 (1998): 33–39.

Duchaine, Dan. "Flavone X: The Next Frontier in Drug Free Muscle Building." *Muscle Media* (May 1996): 64–67.

Friedl, K. E., et al. "Comparison of the Effects of High Dose Testosterone and 19-Nortestoterone to a Replacement Dose of Testosterone on Strength and Body Composition in Normal Men." *Journal of Steroid Biochemistry and Molecular Biology* 40, nos. 4–6 (1991): 607–12.

Gray, A.; Feldman, H.; McKinlay, J.; and Longcope, C. "Age, Disease, and Changing Sex Hormone Levels in Middle-Aged Men: Results of the Massachusetts Male Aging Study." *Journal of Clinical Endocrinology and Metabolism* 73 (1991): 1016–25.

Hanning, Ray V. Jr.; Flood, Charles A.; Hackett, Richard, J.; Loughlin, Jacquelyn, S.; McClure, Neil; and Longcope, Christopher. "Metabolic Clearance Rate of Dehydroepiandrosterone Sulfate, Its Metabolism to Testosterone, and Its Intrafollicular Metabolism to Dehydroepiandrosterone, Androstenedione, Testosterone, and

Dehydrotestosterone in Vivo." *Journal of Clinical Endocrinology and Metabolism.* 72, no. 9 (1991): 1088–94.

Loria, R. M., et al. "Regulation of the Immune Response by Dehydroepiandrosterone and Its Metabolites." *Journal of Endocrinology* 150 (1996): 209–20.

Lowrey, Lonnie, et al. "Conjugated Linoleic Acid Enhances Muscle Size and Strength Gains in Novice Bodybuilders." *Medicine and Science in Sports and Exercise* 30, no. 5 (1998): S182.

Mahesh, V. B., and Greenblatt, R. B. "The In Vivo Conversion of Dehydroepiandrosterone and Androstenedione to Testosterone in the Human." *Aceta Endocrinologica* 41 (1962): 400–06.

Milanov, S. "Effect on the Concentration of Some Hormones in Serum of Healthy Subjects." *Scientific Technical Report.* Sofia, Bulgaria: Chemical Pharmaceutical Institute, 1980.

Sandor, T., and Lanthier, A. "The In Vitro Transformation of 4-Androstene-3, 7-dione to Testosterone by Surviving Human Ovarian Slices." *Canadian Journal of Biochemistry and Physiology* (1960): 445–47.

Seymour-Munn, K., and Adams, J. "Estrogenic Effects of 5-Androstene-3B, 17B-diol at Physiological Concentrations and Its Possible Implication in the Etiology of Breast Cancer." *Endocrinology* 112 (1983): 486–91.

Ullis, Karlis, and Shackman, Joshua. "Androstenedione: The New DHEA." *Nature's Impact* (Apr./May 1998): 21–23.

Vailkov, S. "Apropos of Tribestan Pharmacology." *ScientificTechnical Report.* Sofia, Bulgaria: Chemical Pharmaceutical Institute, 1980.

Wilson, D. Jean, and Foster, W. Daniel. *Williams Textbook of Endocrinology.* Philadelphia, PA: Saunders Company, 1992.

Yen, S. C. *Reproductive Endocrinology.* Philadelphia, PA: Saunders Company, 1978.

Ziegenfuss, Timothy, and Lambert, Lowrey. "Comparison of Androstenedione and 4-Androstenediol and Testostone Levels." Lahti, Finland: International Congress of Weightlifting Training, Nov. 1998.

Chapter 4: How to Lose Fat Naturally

Astrup, A., Buemann, B., Christensen, N. J., Toubro, S., Thorbek, G., Victor, O. J., and Quaade, F. "The Effect of Ephedrine Caffeine Mixture on Energy Metabolism and Body Composition in Obese Women." *Metabolism: Clinical and Experimental* 41, no. 7 (1992): 686–88.

Astrup, A., Toubro, S., Cannon, S., Hein, P., and Madsen, J. "Thermogenic, Metabolic, and Cardiovascular Effects of a Sympathomimetic Agent, Ephedrine." *Current Therapeutic Research* 48, no. 6 (1990): 1087–1100.

Hobbs, Larry S. *The New Diet Pills*. Irvine, CA: Pragmatic Press, 1995.

Leibel, R.; Hirsch, J.; Appel, B. E.; Checani, G. C. "Energy intake required to maintain body weight is not affected by wide variation in diet composition." *American Journal of Clinical Nutrition* 55 (1992): 350–55.

McCarthy, William J. (Letter to the Editor). "Long-Term Maintenance of Weight Loss." *American Journal of Clinical Nutrition* 67 (1998): 946.

O'Sullivan, Anthony, et al. "The Route of Estrogen Replacement Therapy Confers Divergent Effects on Substrate Oxidation and Body Composition in Postmenopausal Women." *The American Society for Clinical Investigation, Journal of Clinical Investigation* 102, no. 5 (Sept. 1998): 1035–40.

Spirduso, W. *Physical Dimensions of Aging*. Champaign, IL: Human Kinetics, 1995.

Stubbs, R. J., et al. "The Effect of Covertly Manipulating the Energy Density of Mixed Diets on Ad Libitum Food Intake in 'Pseudo Free-Living' Humans." *International Journal of Obesity* 22 (1998): 980–87.

Ullis, Karlis, and Ptacek, Greg. *Age Right: Turn Back the Clock with a Proven, Personalized Antiaging Program*. New York: Simon & Schuster, 1999.

Vermeulen, A.; Kaufman, J. M.; and Giagulli, V. A. "Influence of Some Biological Indexes on Sex Hormone Binding Globulin and Androgen Levels in Aging or Obese Males." *Journal of Clinical Endocrinology and Metabolism* 81, no. 5 (1996): 1821–26.

Weigle, D. S. "Human Obesity—Exploding the Myths." *Western Journal of Medicine* 153 (1990): 421–28.

Chapter 5: How to Gain Muscle Naturally

Bhasin, S., and Bremner, William J. "Clinical Review 85: Emerging Issues in Androgen Replacement Therapy." *Journal of Clinical Endocrinology and Metabolism* 82, no. 1 (1997): 3–8.

Bidzinska, B., et al. "Effects of Different Chronic Intermitten Stressors and Acetyl-L-Carnitine on Hypothalamic Beta-Endorphin and GnRH and on Plasma Testosterone in Rats." *Neuroendocrinology* 57 (1993): 985–90.

Dobs, Adrian S., et al. "Pharmacokinetic Characteristics, Efficacy, and Safety of Buccal Testosterone in Hypogonadal Males: A Pilot Study." *Journal of Clinical Endocrinology and Metabolism* 83, no. 1 (1998): 33–39.

Earnest, C. P., et al. "The Effect of Creatine Monohydrate Ingestion on Anaerobic Power Indices, Muscular Strength and Body Composition." *Acta Physiology of Scandinavia* 153 (1995). 207–09.

Fahey, T. D., and Pearl, M. "Hormonal Effects of Phosphatidylserine During Two Weeks of Intense Training." Abstract from National Meeting of the American College of Sports Medicine, June 1998.

Friedl, K., et al. "Comparison of the Effects of High Dose Testosterone and 19-Nortestosterone to a Replacement Dose of Testosterone on Strength and Body Composition in Normal Men." *Journal of Steroid Molecular Biology* 40 (1991): 607–12.

Greenhaff, L., et al. "Influence of Oral Creatine Supplementation on Muscle Torque During Repeated Bouts of Maximal Voluntary Exercise in Man." *Clinical Science* 84 (1993): 565–71.

Hajjar, Ramzi, et al. "Outcomes of Long-Term Testosterone Replacement in Older Hypogonadal Males: A Retrospective Analysis." *Journal of Clinical Endocrinology and Metabolism* 82, no. 11 (1997): 3793–96

Monteleone, P., Maj, M., Beinat, L., Natale, M., and Kemali, D. "Effects of Phosphatidylserine on the Neuroendocrine Response to Physical Stress in Humans." *Neuroendocrinology* 52 (1990): 243–48.

Monteleone, P., Beinat, L., Tanzillo, C., Maj, M., and Kemali, D. "Blunting by Chronic Phosphatidylserine Administration of the Stress-Induced Activation of the Hypothalamo-Pituitary-Adrenal Axis in Healthy Men." *European Journal of Clinical Pharmacology* 43 (1992): 385–88.

Morales, A., et al. "Clinical Practice Guidelines for Screening and Monitoring Male Patients Receiving Testosterone Supplementation Therapy." *International Journal of Impotence Research* 8 (1996): 95–97.

Sih, Rahmawati, et al. "Testosterone Replacement in Older Hypogonadal Men: A 12-Month Randomized Controlled Trial." *Journal of Clinical Endocrinology and Metabolism* 82, no. 6 (1997): 1661–67.

Wadler, G. I., and Hainline, B. *Drugs and the Athlete.* Philadelphia, PA: F. A. Davis, 1989, pp. 55–69.

Chapter 6: The Biochemistry of Sex

Alexander, G., et al. "Androgen Behavior Correlations in Hypogonadal Men and Eugonadal Men. II: Cognitive Abilities." *Hormonal Behavior* 33, no. 2 (Apr. 1998): 85–94.

Anderson-Hunt, Murray, and Dennerstein, Lorraine. "Oxytocin and Female Sexuality." *Gynecology Obstetrics Investigations* 40 (1995): 217–21.

Baskys, A., and Remington, G. *Brain Mechanisms and Psychotropic Drugs.* Boca Raton, FL: CRC Press, 1996, pp. 55–72.

Blum, Deborah. *Sex on the Brain,* New York: Viking, 1997.

Crenshaw, Theresa L. *The Alchemy of Love and Lust.* New York: G. P. Putnam, 1996.

Finkelstein, J. W., et. al. "Effects of Estrogen or Testosterone on Self-Reported Sexual Responses and Behaviors in Hypogonadal Adolescents." *Journal of Clinical Endocrinology and Metabolism* 83, no. 7 (1998): 2281–85.

Fogel, B., and Schiffer, R. *Neuropsychiatry.* Baltimore, MD: Williams and Wilkins, 1996.

Fred, G.; McClure, D.; and Kramer-Levien, D. "Endrocrine Screening for Sexual Dysfunction Using Free Testosterone Determinations." *Journal of Urology* 156 (Aug. 1996): 405–08.

Freud, Sigmund. "Beyond the Pleasure Principle," ed. by James Strachey. New York: W.W. Norton, 1961.

Ganten, D., and Pfaff, D. *Actions of Progesterone on the Brain.* Berlin: Springer-Verlag, 1985.

Henriques, Fernando. *Love in Action.* New York: Dell, 1959.

Kampen, D., and Sherwin, B. "Estradiol Is Related to Visual Memory in Healthy Young Men." *Behavioral Neuroscience* 110, no. 3 (June 1996): 613–17.

Moffat, S., and Hampson, E. "A Curvilinear Relationship Between Testosterone and Spatial Cognition in Humans: Possible Influence of Hand Preference." *Psychoneuroendorcrinology* 21, no. 3 (Apr. 1996): 323–37.

Motta, Marcella. *Brain Endocrinology.* New York: Raven Press, 1991.

Schulkin, Jay. *Hormonally Induced Changes in Mind and Brain.* San Diego, CA: Academic Press, 1993.

Symons, Donald. "Beauty Is in the Adaptions of the Beholder: The Evolutionary Psychology of Human Female Sexual Attractiveness." *Sexual Nature, Sexual Culture,* ed. by Paul R. Abramson and Steven D. Pinkerton, Chicago, IL: University of Chicago Press, 1995.

————. "The Psychology of Human Mate Preferences." *Behavioral and Brain Sciences* 12 (1989): 34–36.

Wallen, Kim. "The Evolution of Female Sexual Desire." *Sexual Nature, Sexual Culture*, ed. by Paul R. Abramson and Steven D. Pinkerton. Chicago, IL: University of Chicago Press, 1995.

Wallen, Kim, and Lovejoy, Jenniffer. "Sexual Behavior: Endocrine Function and Therapy." *Hormonally Induced Changes in Mind and Brain*, ed. by Jay Schulkin. San Diego, CA.: Academic Press, 1993.

Chapter 7: Super T Sexual Cocktails

Alexander, G. M., et al. "Androgen Behavior Correlations in Hypogonadal Men and Eugonadal Men: Mood and Response to Auditory Sexual Stimuli." *Hormonal Behavior* 31, no. 2 (1997): 110–19.

Auger, J., et al. "Decline in Semen Quality Among Fertile Men in Paris During the Past 20 Years." *New England Journal of Medicine* 332 (1995): 281–86.

Aujard, F. "Effect of Vomeronasal Organ Removal on Male Socio-Sexual Responses to Female in a Prosimian Primate (Microcebus Murinus). *Physiology-Behavaior* 62, no. 5 (Nov. 1997): 1003–08.

Bancroft, J., et al. "Androgens and Sexual Behavior in Women Using Oral Contraceptives." *Clinical Endocrinology* 12, no. 4 (Apr. 1980): 327–40.

Buckler, H. M.; Robertson, W. R.; and Wu, F.C.W. "Which Androgen Replacement Therapy for Women?" *Journal of Clinical Endocrinology and Metabolism* 83, no. 11 (1998): 3920–24.

Crenshaw, Theresa L., M.D., and Goldberg, James P., Ph.D. *Sexual Pharmacology: Drugs That Affect Sexual Functioning*. New York: W. W. Norton, 1996.

Dennerstein, Lorraine, et al. "Sexuality, Hormones, and the Menopausal Tradition." *Maturitas* 26 (1997): 83–93.

Kaplan, Helen Singer, M.D., Ph.D. *The New Sex Therapy: Active Treatment of Sexual Dysfunctions*. New York: Brunner/Mazel Publications, 1974.

Karavolas, H., and Hodges, D. R. "Neuroendocrine Metabolism of Progesterone and Related Progestins." *Steroids and Neuronal Activity*. New York: John Wiley, 1990.

Kuiper, George G.J.M., et al. "Estrogen Is a Male and Female Hormone." *Science and Medicine* 5, no. 4 (1998): 36–45.

Labrie, F., et al. "Marked Decline in Serum Concentrations of Adrenal C19 Sex Steroid Precursors and Conjugated Androgen

Metabolites During Aging." *Journal of Clinical Endocrinology and Metabolism* 82, no. 6 (1998): 2396–2402.

Morales, Arlene J., et al. "Effects of Replacement Dose of Dehydroepiandrosterone in Men and Women of Advancing Age." *Journal of Endocrinology and Metabolism* 78, no. 6 (1994): 1360–67.

Mortola, J. F. and Yen, S.S.C. "The Effects of Oral Dehydroepiandrosterone on Endocrine-Metalbolic Parameters in Postmenopausal Women." *Journal of Clinical Endocrinology and Metabolism* 71, no. 3 (1990): 696–703.

Moss, R. L., et al. "Urine Derived Compound Evokes Membrane Responses in Mouse Vomeronasal Receptor Neurons." *Journal of Neurophysiology* 77, no. 5 (1997): 2856–62.

Sherins, R. J. "Are Semen Quality and Male Fertility Changing?" *New England Journal of Medicine* 332 (1995): 327.

Tricker, R., et al. "The Effects of Supraphysiological Doses of Testosterone on Angry Behavior in Healthy Eugonadal Men: A Clinical Research Center Study." *Journal of Clinical Endocrinology and Metabolism* 81, no. 10 (Oct. 1996): 3754–58.

Van Goozen, Stephanie H. M., Ph.D., et al. "Psychoendocrinological Assessment of the Menstrual Cycle: The Relationship Between Hormones, Sexuality, and Mood." *Archives of Sexual Behavior* 26, no. 4 (1997): 359–82.

Wang, C., et al. "Testosterone Replacement Therapy Improves Mood in Hypogonadal Men. A Clinical Research Center Study." *Journal of Clinical Endocrinology and Metabolism* 81, no. 10 (Oct. 1996): 3578–83.

Wilcox, A. J., et al. "Fertility in Men Exposed Prenatally to Diethylstilbestrol." *New England Journal of Medicine* 332 (1995): 1411–16.

Chapter 8: Pro-Sexual Lifestyle Strategies

Anderson, K. E., et al. "Diet-Hormone Interactions: Protein Carbohydrate Ratio Relates Reciprocally to the Plasma Levels of Testosterone and Cortisol and Their Respective Binding Globulins in Man." *Life Sciences* 40 (1987): 1761–68.

Belanger, A. et al. "Influence of Diet on Plasma Steroids and Sex Hormone-Binding Globulin Levels in Adult Men." *Journal of Steroid Biochemistry* 32, no. 6 (1989): 829–33.

Chia, Mantak, and Winn, Michael. *Taoist Secrets of Love: Cultivating Male Sexual Energy*. New York: Aurora Press, 1984.

Dorgan, J. F. "Relation of Energy, Fat and Fiber Intakes to Plasma Concentrations of Estrogens and Androgens in Premenopausal Women." *American Journal of Clinical Nutrition* 64, no. 1 (1996): 25–31.

Erasmus, Udo. *Fats and Oils: The Complete Guide to Fats and Oils in Health and Nutrition.* Vancouver, Canada: Alive Books, 1986.

Goldin, B. R., et al. "The Effect of Dietary Fat and Fiber on Serum Estrogen Concentrations in Premenopausal Women Under Controlled Dietary Conditions." *Cancer* 74, no. 3 Suppl. (1994): 1125–31.

Gray, A., et al. "Age, Disease, and Changing Sex Hormone Levels in Middle-Aged Men: Results of the Massachusetts Male Aging Study." *Journal of Clinical Endocrinology and Metabolism* 73, no. 5 (1991): 1016–25.

Haavio, Mannila E., and Kontula, O. "Correlates of Increased Sexual Satisfaction." *Arch-Sex-Behav.* 26, no. 4 (1997): 399–419.

Lieber, C. S., "Hepatic and Metabolic Effects of Ethanol: Pathogenesis and Prevention." *Annals of Internal Medicine* 26, no. 5 (1994): 325–30.

Raben, A., et al. "Sex Hormones and Endurance Performance After a Lacto-Ovo Vegetarian and a Mixed Diet." *Medicine and Science in Sports and Exercise* 24, no. 11 (1992): 1290–97.

Rosler, Ariel, M.D., and Witztum, Eliezer, M.D. "Treatment of Men with Paraphilia with a Long-Acting Analogue of Gonadotropin-Releasing Hormone." *New England Journal of Medicine* (Feb. 1998): 416–65.

Simopoulos, Artemis P., M.D., and Robinson, Jo. *The Omega Plan: The Medically Proven Diet That Gives You the Essential Nutrients You Need.* New York: HarperCollins, 1998.

Tham, D., et al. "Potential Health Benefits of Dietary Phytoestrogens: A Review of the Clinical, Epidemiological and Mechanistic Evidence." *Journal of Clinical Endocrinology and Metabolism* 83, no. 7 (1998): 2223–35.

Volek, J., et al. "Testosterone and Cortisol in Relationship to Dietary Nutrients and Resistance Exercise." *Journal of Applied Physiology* 82, no. 1 (Jan. 1997): 49–54.

Wenz, M., et al. "Substrate Oxidation at Rest and During Exercise: Effects of Menstrual Cycle Phase and Diet Composition." *Journal of Physiology Pharmacology* 48, no. 4 (1997): 851–60.

Chapter 10: Medicine Chest

Carper, Jean. *Miracle Cures*. New York: HarperCollins, 1997.

Hobbs, Larry S. *The New Diet Pills*. Irvine, CA: Pragmatic Press 1995.

Lowrey, Lonnie, et al. "Conjugated Linoleic Acid Enhances Muscle Size and Strength Gains in Novice Bodybuilders." *Medicine and Science in Sports and Exercise* 30.5 (1998): S182.

Meikle, Wayne A., et al. "Effects of Fat-Containing Meal on Sex Hormones in Men." *Journal of Endocrinology and Metabolism* 39, no. 9 (Sept. 1990): 943–46.

Murray, Michael T. *Encyclopedia of Nutritional Supplements*. Rocklin, CA: Prima Publishing, 1996.

Werbach, Melvyn R. *Nutritional Influences on Illness*. Tarzana, CA: Third Line Press, 1996.

————, and Murray, Michael T. *Botanical Influences on Illness*. Tarzana, CA: Third Line Press, 1994.

Ziegenfuss, Timothy, and Lambert, Lowrey. "Comparison of Androstenedione and 4-Androstenediol and Testostone Levels." Lahti, Finland: International Congress of Weightlifting Training, Nov. 1998.

Appendix 2: Sex-Busting Drugs

Lamm, Steven, M.D., and Couzens, Gerald Secor. *The Virility Solution*. New York: Simon & Schuster, 1998.

Appendix 3: Exercise

Douglas, Nik, and Slinger, Penny. *Sexual Secrets the Alchemy of Ecstacy*. New York: Destiny Books, 1979.

Mookerjee, Ajit. *Kundalini: The Arousal of the Inner Energy*. Rochester, NY: Vermont Destiny Books, 1991.

Phelan, Nancy, and Volin, Michael. *Sex and Yoga*. New York: Bantam, 1968.

Yogiraj Sri Swami Satchidananda. *Integral Yoga Hatha*. New York: Holt, Rinehart and Winston, 1970.

⋆ Index ⋆

•⊷ About the Author ⊷•

KARLIS ULLIS, M.D., is the founder and medical director of the Sports Medicine and Anti-Aging Medical Group in Santa Monica, California. This full-service clinic specializes in advanced antiaging medicine, hormone replacement (menopause and andropause), fitness and weight-loss programs, growth hormone therapies, physical rehabilitation, and antiaging skin diagnostics and treatment. The center also conducts antiaging research and product development. For more information call 310-829-1990 or fax 310-829-5134.

Dr. Ullis's prosexual and antiaging formulas are now available to the public.

For more information visit his Website at http://www.agingprevent.com.